Urological Emergencies
in Clinical Practice

Hashim Hashim • John Reynard
Nigel C. Cowan • Dan Wood
Noel Armenakas
Editors

Urological Emergencies in Clinical Practice

Second Edition

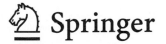 Springer

Editors

Hashim Hashim
Consultant Urological Surgeon and
Director of the Urodynamics Unit
Department of Urology
Bristol Urological Institute
Southmead Hospital, Bristol, UK

John Reynard
Department of Urology, Nuffield
Department of Surgical Sciences
Oxford University Hospitals
Oxford, UK

The National Spinal Injuries Centre
Stoke Mandeville Hospital
Aylesbury, UK

Nigel C. Cowan
Department of Radiology
The Churchill Hospital
Oxford, UK

Dan Wood
Department of Adolescent
and Reconstructive Urology
University College London
Hospitals, London, UK

Department of Urology
Great Ormond Street Hospital
London, UK

University College London
London, UK

Noel Armenakas
Department of Urology
Lenox Hill Hospital and New York
Presbyterian Hospital (Cornell-Weill)
New York, NY, USA

ISBN 978-1-4471-2719-2   ISBN 978-1-4471-2720-8   (eBook)
DOI 10.1007/978-1-4471-2720-8
Springer London Heidelberg New York Dordrecht

Library of Congress Control Number: 2013932850

Contents

Chapter 1
Presenting Symptoms of Urological Emergencies

Hashim Hashim

Flank Pain

Flank pain is regarded as a classic symptom of renal or ureteric pathology. Indeed, it is often immediately assumed that a patient who presents with flank pain has a stone in the ureter or kidney. However, only 50% of patients who present with flank pain have a ureteric stone confirmed on imaging studies (Smith et al. 1996; Thomson et al. 2001). The other 50% have non-stone-related disease (and more often than not, non-urological disease), the differential diagnosis of which is long and dependent on the age, the side of the pain, and the sex of the patient.

The multiple causes of flank pain, to an extent, reflect the fact that the nerve roots subserving pain sensation from the kidney also subserve pain sensation from other organs. Pain sensation from the kidney primarily is transmitted via preganglionic sympathetic nerves that reach spinal cord levels T11 to L2 through the dorsal nerve roots. These same nerve roots supply pain fibers to other intra-abdominal organs. Similarly, pain derived from the T10 to T12 costal nerves can also be confused with renal colic.

H. Hashim, M.D., FEBU, FRCS (Urol)
Consultant Urological Surgeon and Director of the Urodynamics Unit,
Department of Urology, Bristol Urological Institute,
Southmead Hospital, Bristol, UK
e-mail: h.hashim@gmail.com

H. Hashim et al. (eds.), *Urological Emergencies*
In Clinical Practice, DOI 10.1007/978-1-4471-2720-8_1,
© Springer-Verlag London 2013

Causes

This list of causes of flank pain is not exhaustive. Some of these alternative causes may seem bizarre, but we have seen examples of all of these conditions, which were initially referred to us as "ureteric stone pain," but where the final diagnosis was some other cause.

Pain on Either Side

- Urological causes: ureteric stones, renal stones, renal or ureteric tumors, renal infection (pyelonephritis, perinephric abscess, pyonephrosis), pelviureteric junction obstruction
- Medical causes of flank pain: myocardial infarction, pneumonia, rib fracture, malaria, pulmonary embolus
- Gynecological and obstetric disease: twisted ovarian cysts, ectopic pregnancy, salpingitis
- Other non-urological causes: pancreatitis, diverticulitis, inflammatory bowel disease, peptic ulcer disease, gastritis

Right-Side Flank Pain

- Biliary colic, cholecystitis, hepatitis, appendicitis

When flank pain has a urological origin, it occurs as a consequence of distention of the renal capsule by inflammatory or neoplastic disease (pain of constant intensity) or as a consequence of obstruction to the kidney (pain of fluctuating intensity). In the case of ureteric obstruction by a stone, pain also arises as a consequence of obstruction to the kidney and from localized inflammation within the ureter.

Characteristics of flank pain due to ureteric stones: this pain is typically of sudden onset, located below the costovertebral angle of the twelfth rib and lateral to the sacrospinalis muscle, and it radiates anteriorly to the abdomen and inferiorly to the ipsilateral groin. The intensity may increase rapidly, reaching a peak within minutes or may increase more slowly over the course of 1–2 h. The patient cannot get comfortable and tries to move in an attempt to relieve the pain. The pain is not exacerbated by movement or posture. Associated symptoms, occurring with variable frequency include nausea, vomiting, and hematuria.

Patients with pathology that irritates the peritoneum (i.e., peritonitis) usually lie motionless/still. Any movement, or palpation, exacerbates the pain. Patients with renal colic try to move around to find a more comfortable position. The pain may radiate to the shoulder tip or scapula if there is irritation of the diaphragm (the sensory innervation of which is by the phrenic nerve, spinal nerve root C4). Shoulder-tip pain is not a feature of urological disease.

Hematuria

While hematuria is only relatively rarely an emergency (presenting as clot retention, clot colic, or anemia), it is such an alarming symptom that it may cause a patient to present to the emergency department.

Blood in the urine may be seen with the naked eye (variously described as macroscopic, frank, or gross hematuria) or may be detected on urine dipstick (dipstick hematuria) or by microscopic examination of urine (microscopic hematuria, defined as the presence of >3 red blood cells per high-power microscopic field). Just 5 mL of blood in 1 L of urine is visible with the naked eye. Dipstick tests, for blood in the urine, test for hemoglobin rather than intact red blood cells. A cause for the hematuria cannot be found in a substantial proportion of patients despite investigations in the form of flexible cystoscopy, renal ultrasonography, intravenous urography (IVU), or computed tomogram urography (CTU). No cause for the hematuria is found in approximately 50% of patients with macroscopic hematuria and 60–70% of patients with microscopic hematuria (Khadra et al. 2000).

Hematuria has nephrological (medical) or urological (surgical) causes. Medical causes are glomerular and non-glomerular, for example, blood dyscrasias, interstitial nephritis, and renovascular disease. Glomerular hematuria results in dysmorphic erythrocytes (distorted during their passage through the glomerulus), red blood cell casts, and proteinuria, while non-glomerular hematuria (bleeding from a site in the nephron distal to the glomerulus) results in circular erythrocytes, the absence of erythrocyte casts, and the absence of proteinuria.

Surgical/urological non-glomerular causes include renal tumors, urothelial tumors (bladder, ureteric, renal collecting system), prostate cancer, bleeding from vascular benign prostatic enlargement, trauma, renal or ureteric stones, and urinary tract infection. Hematuria in these situations is usually characterized by circular erythrocytes and absence of proteinuria and casts.

Hematuria can be painless or painful. It can occur at the beginning of the urinary stream, at the end of the urinary stream, or be present throughout the stream. Hematuria at the beginning of the stream may indicate urethral or prostatic pathology. Hematuria at the end of the stream may indicate prostatic urethra or bladder neck pathology, and that present throughout the stream of urine may indicate renal or bladder pathology.

Associated symptoms help determine the cause. Associated renal angle pain suggests a renal or ureteric source for the hematuria, whereas suprapubic pain suggests a bladder source. Painless frank hematuria is not infrequently due to bladder cancer.

As stated above, while patients sometimes present acutely to their family doctors or to hospital emergency departments with hematuria, it is seldom a urological emergency, unless the bleeding is so heavy that the patient has become anemic as a consequence (this is rare) or the bladder or a ureter has become blocked by clots (in which case, the patient presents with retention of urine or with ureteric colic, which may mimic that due to a stone).

We investigate all patients with hematuria and recommend, as a bare minimum, urine culture and cytology, renal ultrasonography, and flexible cystoscopy, with more complex investigations such as an IVU or CTU in selected groups.

Anuria, Oliguria, and Inability to Pass Urine

Anuria is defined as complete absence of urine production and usually indicates obstruction to the urinary tract. The level of obstruction may be at the outlet of the bladder or at the level of the ureters bilaterally. Unrelieved bilateral urinary tract obstruction leads rapidly to acute renal failure, which may have very serious consequences (e.g., hyperkalemia, fluid overload).

If the level of obstruction is at the outlet of the bladder, abdominal examination will reveal a percussable and palpably distended bladder. Urine will be present in the bladder on catheterization, and urine output will resume once a catheter has bypassed the obstruction. The commonest cause is benign prostatic enlargement and less commonly malignant enlargement of the prostate.

If the obstruction is at the level of the lower ureters or ureteric orifices, the bladder will not be palpable or percussable. Catheterization will reveal no, or a very low, volume of urine in the bladder, and there will be no improvement in urine output or of renal function post-catheterization. Causes include locally advanced prostate cancer, extensive involvement of the trigone of the bladder by bladder cancer, and locally advanced cervical or rectal cancer. Rectal or vaginal examination may reveal a cervical, prostatic, or rectal cancer, and cystoscopic examination of the bladder may demonstrate a bladder cancer.

Bilateral obstruction higher up the ureters may be due to extensive lymph node metastases to the pelvic and para-aortic nodes from distant malignancy, retroperitoneal fibrosis, and rarely bilateral ureteric stones. Evidence of a malignancy elsewhere may be found on clinical examination. The diagnosis is usually made on the basis of excluding obstruction at the outlet of the bladder and in the lower ureters and by radiographic imaging (ultrasound and abdominal CT).

Oliguria is scanty urine production and more precisely is defined as urine production of less than 400 mL/day in adults and less than 1 mL/kg of bodyweight per hour in children. The causes are prerenal (e.g., hypovolemia, hypotension), renal (e.g., acute vasculitis, acute glomerular lesions, acute interstitial nephritis, and acute tubular necrosis from nephrotoxic drugs, toxins, or sepsis), and postrenal causes (as for anuria, but where the degree of obstruction has not yet reached a level critical enough to stop urine production completely).

Suprapubic Pain

Suprapubic pain can be caused by overdistention of the bladder and inflammatory, infective, and neoplastic conditions of the bladder. All such conditions may present as an emergency. Bladder overdistention may result from bladder outflow obstruction, for example, by an enlarged prostate or urethral stricture. Painful inability to empty the bladder is defined as urinary retention.

Urinary tract infection is usually associated with urethral burning or scalding on voiding; frequent, low-volume voiding; and a feeling of incomplete bladder emptying with an immediate desire to void again. The urine may be offensive to smell.

Inflammatory conditions of the bladder such as interstitial cystitis can also cause suprapubic pain, as can carcinoma in-situ. Gynecological causes of suprapubic pain include endometriosis, fibroids, and ovarian pathology. Gastrointestinal causes of suprapubic pain include inflammatory and neoplastic bowel disease and irritable bowel syndrome.

Scrotal Pain and Swelling

Scrotal pain may arise as a consequence of pathology within the scrotum itself (e.g., torsion of the testicles or its appendages, epididymo-orchitis), or it may be referred from disease elsewhere (e.g., the pain of ureteric colic may be referred to the testis).

The classic presentation of testicular torsion is one of sudden onset of acute pain in the hemi-scrotum, sometimes waking the patient from sleep. It may radiate to the groin and/or the loin. There may be a history of mild trauma to the testis in the hours before the acute onset of pain. Similar episodes may have occurred in the past, with spontaneous resolution of the pain, suggesting torsion with spontaneous detorsion. Patients will be in considerable pain. They may have a slight fever. They do not like the testis being touched and will find it difficult to walk and to get up on the examination couch, as movement exacerbates the pain. The testis is usually swollen, very tender to touch, and may appear abnormally tense (if the patient lets you squeeze it!). It may be high riding (lying at a higher than normal position in the scrotum) and may lie horizontally due to twisting of the cord with difficulty in feeling the cord. The testis may feel hard, and there may be scrotal wall erythema.

Epididymo-orchitis may present with similar symptoms. The localization of tenderness in the epididymis and the absence of testicular tenderness may help to distinguish epididymo-orchitis from testicular torsion, but in many cases, it is difficult to make a precise diagnosis on clinical grounds alone, and often testicular exploration is the only way of establishing the diagnosis with certainty.

Other scrotal pathology may present as acute scrotal swelling leading to emergency presentation. Rarely testicular tumors present as an emergency with rapid onset (days) of scrotal swelling. Very rarely they present with advanced metastatic disease (see Chap. 9).

Priapism

Priapism is a painful persistent prolonged erection not related to sexual stimulation. Its causes are summarized in Chap. 6. Knowledge of these causes allows appropriate questions to be asked during history taking. The two broad categories of priapism are low-flow (most common) and high-flow. Low-flow priapism is essentially due to hemato-logical disease, malignant infiltration of the corpora cavern-osa with malignant disease, or drugs. High-flow priapism is due to perineal trauma, which creates an arteriovenous fistula. It is painless, unlike low-flow priapism, where ischemia of the erectile tissue causes pain.

The diagnosis of priapism is usually obvious from the history and examination of the erect, tender penis (in low-flow priapism). Characteristically, the corpora cavernosa are rigid, and the glans is flaccid. Examine the abdomen for evidence of malignant disease and perform a digital rectal examination to examine the prostate and check anal tone.

Back Pain and Urological Symptoms

Occasionally, patients with urological disease present with associated back pain. In some cases, this may be the very first symptom of urological disease, and it may be so severe that the patient may present acutely to the emergency department. In general terms, there are two broad categories of disease that may present with back pain and urological symptoms: neurological conditions and malignant conditions of urological or non-urological origin.

Neurological Disease

Patients with neurological disease may present with both back pain and disturbed lower urinary tract, disturbed bowel, and disturbed sexual function. Such conditions include spinal cord and cauda equina tumors and prolapsed intervertebral discs. In all of these conditions, back pain is the most common early presenting symptom. It is usually gradual in onset and progresses slowly but relentlessly. Associated symptoms suggestive of a neurological cause for the pain include pins and needles in the hands or feet, weakness in the arms (cervical cord) or legs (lumbosacral spine), urinary symptoms such as hesitancy and a poor urinary flow, constipation, loss of erections, and seemingly bizarre symptoms, such as loss of sensation of orgasm or absent ejaculation. From time to time, the patient may present in urinary retention. It is all too easy to assume that this is due to prostatic obstruction if a focused neurological history is not sought and a focused neurological examination is not performed.

Malignant Disease

Malignant tumors may metastasize to the vertebral column, where they may compress the spinal cord (spinal cord compression) or the nerve roots that comprise the cauda equina. Examples include urological malignancies such as prostate cancer and non-urological malignancies such as lung cancer. In so doing, they may cause both back pain and disturbed urinary, bowel, and sexual function. The pain of vertebral metastases may be localized to the area of the involved vertebra but may also involve adjacent spinal nerve roots, causing radicular pain. Interscapular pain that wakes the patient at night is characteristic of a metastatic deposit in the thoracic spine.

The physical sign of spinal cord compression is a sensory level, but this tends to occur late in the day in the course of the condition. Remember, however, that a normal neurological examination does not exclude a diagnosis of cord compression. If, on the basis of the patient's symptoms, you suspect cord compression, arrange for a magnetic resonance imaging (MRI) scan without delay.

Malignant infiltration of retroperitoneal lymph nodes by, for example, testicular cancers or lymphoma can also cause back pain.

As a general rule, if a patient presents with bizarre symptoms that are difficult to explain, consider the possibility of a neurological cause.

References

Khadra MH, Pickard RS, Charlton M, et al. A prospective analysis of 1,930 patients with hematuria to evaluate current diagnostic practice. J Urol. 2000;163:524–7.

Smith RC, Verga M, McCarthy S, Rosenfield AT. Diagnosis of acute flank pain: value of unenhanced helical CT. AJR Am J Roentgenol. 1996;166:97–101.

Thomson JM, Glocer J, Abbott C, ct al. Computed tomography versus intravenous urography in diagnosis of acute flank pain from urolithiasis: a randomized study comparing imaging costs and radiation dose. Australas Radiol. 2001;45:291–7.

Chapter 2
Lower Urinary Tract Emergencies

John Reynard

Acute Urinary Retention

Definition

Painful inability to void, with relief of pain following drainage of the bladder by catheterization.

The combination of reduced or absent urine output with lower abdominal pain is not in itself enough to make a diagnosis of acute retention. Many acute surgical conditions cause abdominal pain and fluid depletion, the latter leading to reduced urine output, and this reduced urine output can give the erroneous impression that the patient is in retention, when in fact they are not. Thus, central to the diagnosis is the presence of a *large* volume of urine, which when drained by

J. Reynard, DM, FRCS (Urol)
Department of Urology, Nuffield Department of Surgical Sciences, Oxford University Hospitals, Oxford, UK

The National Spinal Injuries Centre, Stoke Mandeville Hospital, Aylesbury, UK
e-mail: john.reynard@ouh.nhs.uk

H. Hashim et al. (eds.), *Urological Emergencies*
In Clinical Practice, DOI 10.1007/978-1-4471-2720-8_2,
© Springer-Verlag London 2013

catheterization, leads to resolution of the pain. What represents "large" has not been strictly defined, but volumes of 500–800 mL are typical. Volumes <500 mL should lead one to question the diagnosis. Volumes >800 mL are defined as acute-on-chronic retention (see section Is It Acute or Chronic Retention?).

Pathophysiology

There are three broad mechanisms:

- Increased urethral *resistance*, i.e., bladder outlet obstruction (BOO)
- Low bladder *pressure*, i.e., impaired bladder contractility
- Interruption of sensory or motor innervation of the bladder

Causes in Men

The commonest cause is benign prostatic enlargement (BPE) due to benign prostatic hyperplasia (BPH) leading to BOO; less common causes include malignant enlargement of the prostate, urethral stricture, and, rarely, prostatic abscess.

Urinary retention in men is either *spontaneous* (usually being preceded by the presence of lower urinary tract symptoms), *precipitated by an event* in a previously asymptomatic patient or be precipitated by an event in a previously symptomatic patient. Precipitated retention is less likely to recur once the event that caused it has been removed. Spontaneous retention is more likely to recur after a trial of catheter removal, and therefore is more likely to require definitive treatment, e.g., transurethral resection of the prostate (TURP). Precipitating events include anesthetics and other drugs (anticholinergics, sympathomimetic agents such as ephedrine in nasal decongestants), non-prostatic abdominal or perineal surgery, and immobility following surgical procedures, e.g., total hip replacement.

Causes in Women

There are more possible causes in women, but acute urinary retention is less common than it is in men. The causes include pelvic prolapse (cystocele, rectocele, uterine), the prolapsing organ directly compressing the urethra; urethral stricture; urethral diverticulum; postsurgery for "stress" incontinence; Fowler's syndrome (impaired relaxation of external sphincter occurring in premenopausal women, often in association with polycystic ovaries); and pelvic masses (e.g., ovarian masses) (Fowler 2003). Postpartum retention is discussed below.

Causes in Either Sex

A wide variety of pathologies can cause urinary retention in both men and women: hematuria leading to clot retention, drugs (as above), pain (adrenergic stimulation of the bladder neck), postoperative retention, sacral (S2–S4) nerve compression or damage—so-called cauda equina compression (due to prolapsed L2–L3 disk or L3–L4 intervertebral disk, trauma to the vertebrae, benign or metastatic tumors), radical pelvic surgery damaging the parasympathetic plexus (radical hysterectomy, abdominoperineal resection), pelvic fracture rupturing the urethra (more likely in men than women), neurotropic viruses involving the sensory dorsal root ganglia of S2–S4 (herpes simplex or zoster), multiple sclerosis, transverse myelitis, diabetic cystopathy, and damage to dorsal columns of spinal cord causing loss of bladder sensation (tabes dorsalis, pernicious anemia).

Neurological Causes of Retention: A Word of Warning!

It is all too easy to assume that urinary retention in a man is due to BPE. Of course this is by far the commonest cause in elderly men, but in the younger man (below the age of 60, but even in some men older than 60), spend a few moments considering whether there might be some other cause. Similarly, in women, where retention is much less common than in men, think *why* the patient went into retention.

Be wary of the patient with a history of constipation and be particularly wary where there is associated back pain. We all get back pain from time to time, but pain of neurological origin, such as that due to a spinal tumor or due to cauda equina compression from a prolapsed intervertebral disk (pressing on S2–S4 nerve roots, thereby impairing bladder contraction), may be severe, relentless, and progressive. The patient may say that the pain has become severe in the weeks before the episode of retention. Nighttime back pain and sciatica (pain shooting down the back of the thigh and legs), which are relieved by sitting in a chair or by pacing around the bedroom at night, are typical of the pain caused by a neurofibroma or ependymoma affecting the cauda equina. Interscapular back pain is typically caused by tumors that have metastasized to the thoracic spine.

Altered sensation due to a cauda equina compression can manifest as the inability to tell whether the bladder is full, inability to feel urine passing down their urethra while voiding, and difficulty in knowing whether one is going to pass feces or flatus.

Male patients with a neurological cause for their retention (such as spinal tumor) may report symptoms of sexual dysfunction that may appear bizarre (and may therefore be dismissed). They might have lost the ability to get an erection or have lost the sensation of orgasm. They might complain of odd burning or tingling sensations in the perineum or penis.

It does not take more than a minute or two to ask a few relevant questions (Are you constipated? Have you had back pain? Do your legs feel funny or weak?), to establish on examination whether the patient has a sensory level (the cardinal sign of a cord compression), to test for other neurological signs of a cord compression, and to test the integrity of the sacral nerve roots that subserve bladder function—S2–S4. In the male patient, this can be done by squeezing the glans of the penis while performing a digital rectal examination (DRE). Contraction of the anus, felt by the physician's palpating finger, indicates that the afferent and efferent sacral nerves and the sacral cord are intact. This is the bulbocavernosus reflex (BCR). In women, once catheterized, the "same" reflex can be elicited by gently tugging the catheter onto the bladder neck, again while doing a DRE. Again, contraction of the anus indicates that the afferent and efferent sacral nerves and the sacral cord are intact.

If you do not know about these rare causes of retention, you would not think to ask the relevant questions. Missing the diagnosis in such cases can have profound implications for the patient (and for you). One should have a low threshold for arranging an urgent magnetic resonance imaging (MRI) scan of the thoracic, lumbar, and sacral cord and of the cauda equina in patients who present in urinary retention with these additional symptoms or signs.

Risk Factors for Postoperative Retention

Postoperative retention may be precipitated by instrumentation of the lower urinary tract, surgery to the perineum or anorectum, gynecological surgery, bladder overdistention, reduced sensation of bladder fullness, preexisting prostatic obstruction, and epidural anesthesia. Postpartum urinary retention is not uncommon, particularly with epidural anesthesia and instrumental delivery.

Urinary Retention: Initial Management

Urethral catheterization is the mainstay of initial management of urinary retention. This relieves the pain of the overdistended bladder. If it is not possible to pass a catheter urethrally, then a suprapubic catheter will be required. Record the volume drained—this confirms the diagnosis, determines subsequent management, and provides prognostic information with regard to outcome from this treatment.

Is It Acute or Chronic Retention?

There is a group of elderly men who are in urinary retention, but who are not aware of it. This is so-called high-
pressure chronic retention. Mitchell (1984) defined
high-pressure chronic retention of urine as maintenance of
voiding, with a bladder volume of >800 mL and an intravesical
pressure above 30 cm H_2O, often accompanied by hydronephrosis (Abrams et al. 1978; George et al. 1983). Over
time, this leads to renal failure. The patient continues to
void spontaneously and will often have no sensation of
incomplete emptying. His bladder seems to be insensitive to
the gross distention. Often, the first presenting symptom is
bed-wetting. This is such an unpleasant and disruptive
symptom that it will cause most people to visit their doctor.
In such cases, inspection of the abdomen will show gross
distention of the bladder, which may be confirmed by palpation and percussion of the tense bladder.

Sometimes the patient with high-pressure chronic retention is suddenly unable to pass urine, and in this situation,
so-called acute-on-chronic high-pressure retention of urine
has developed.

On catheterization, a large volume of urine is drained
from the bladder (often in the order of 1–2 L and sometimes
much greater). The serum creatinine will be elevated, and an
ultrasound will show hydronephrosis (Fig. 2.1) with a grossly
distended bladder.

Recording the volume of urine obtained following catheterization can help define two groups of patients, those with
acute retention of urine (retention volume <800 mL) and
those with acute-on-chronic retention (retention volume
>800 mL). Prior to catheterization, if the patient reports
recent bed-wetting, you may suspect that you are dealing
with a case of high-pressure acute-on-chronic retention. The
retention volume will confirm the diagnosis.

Where the patient has a high retention volume (more than
a couple of liters), the serum creatinine is elevated, and a
renal ultrasound shows hydronephrosis, anticipate that a

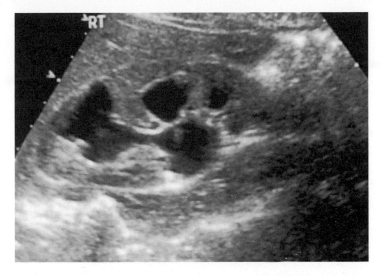

FIGURE 2.1 Hydronephrosis in a case of high-pressure chronic retention

post-obstructive diuresis is going to occur. This can be very marked and is due to a number of factors:

- Reduction in urine flow through the loop of Henle removes the "driving force" behind development of the corticomedullary concentration gradient. In addition, continued perfusion of the kidney effectively also "washes out" this gradient, which is essential for allowing the kidney to concentrate urine. Once normal flow through the nephron has recommenced following emptying of the bladder and removal of the back pressure on the kidney, it takes a few days for this corticomedullary concentration gradient to be reestablished. During this period, the kidney cannot concentrate the urine, and a diuresis occurs until the corticomedullary concentration gradient is reestablished.
- The elevated serum urea acts as an osmotic diuretic.
- Excessive salt and water, laid down during the period of retention, is appropriately excreted by the kidney.

Usually the patient comes to no harm from this diuresis, even when several liters of urine are excreted per 24 h. However, occasionally the intravascular volume may fall, and postural hypotension may develop. One good way of anticipating this is to record lying and standing blood pressure. If there is a large discrepancy between the two, consider intravenous fluid replacement with normal saline.

What to Do Next for the Man with Acute Retention

Precipitated retention often does not recur. Spontaneous retention often does.

Precipitated urinary retention should be managed by a trial of catheter removal. In spontaneous retention, many urologists will try to avoid proceeding straight to transurethral resection of the prostate (TURP) after just one episode of retention, instead recommending a trial of catheter removal, with or without an alpha-blocker, in the hope that the patient will void spontaneously and avoid the need for operation. A trial without catheter is clearly not appropriate in cases where there is back pressure on the kidneys—high-pressure retention. About a quarter of men with acute retention will void successfully after a trial without catheter (Djavan et al. 1997; Hastie et al. 1990). Of those who pass urine successfully after an initial episode of retention, about 50 % will go back into retention within a week, 60 % within a month, and 70 % after a year. This means that after 1 year, only about one in 5–10 men originally presenting with urinary retention will not have gone back into retention. Recurrent retention is more likely in those with a flow rate <5 mL/s or average voided volumes of <150 mL. An alpha-blocker started 24 h before a trial of catheter removal increases the chances of voiding successfully (30 % taking placebo voiding successfully, and 50 % taking an alpha-blocker doing so; McNeill et al. 1999). However, whether continued use of an alpha-blocker after an episode of acute retention reduces the risk of a further episode of retention (McNeill 2001) is not yet known.

So, a trial of an alpha-blocker is reasonable, but a substantial number of men with spontaneous acute retention of urine will end up going back into retention and will therefore eventually come under the care of a urologist for TURP.

Retention in Patients with a Catheterizable Stoma

An increasing number of patients have undergone reconstructive surgery involving the formation of a catheterizable stoma, such as a Mitrofanoff stoma.

Patients with a Mitrofanoff catheterizable stoma are sometimes unable to pass a catheter into their stoma. This not infrequently occurs after spinal or other surgery. The spinal surgery may change the "angle" of the stoma or their bladder may become overfull in the postoperative period which again may distort the stoma to the extent that it is difficult to pass a catheter. In this situation:

(a) Attempt to pass the catheter yourself; using plenty of lubrication is reasonable. If the patient's usual size catheter will not pass, go up or down a size.

(b) If you fail, try to pass a floppy guidewire through the stoma (preferably under radiological control if this is available). This may pass into the bladder where the catheter will not. A catheter, with the tip cut off, can then be passed over the guidewire and into the bladder.

(c) If this fails, consider passing a flexible ureterorenoscope (a flexible cystoscope if often too large) as far as possible over a guidewire and attempt to negotiate a route into the bladder.

(d) If all else fails, pass a suprapubic catheter and empty the bladder, and then usually the patient will be able to pass their catheter without any problems.

Postpartum Retention of Urine

Postpartum urinary retention is the inability to void spontaneously after delivery. Beyond this basic definition, there is a lack of an agreed definition of retention both in terms of either the time of onset or the bladder volume at the time of retention.

A definition for postpartum urinary retention that has been used (Yip 2004) is the absence of spontaneous micturition within 6 h of vaginal delivery (in case of a cesarean section, 6 h after the removal of the bladder catheter). While this is a somewhat arbitrary[1] definition, concordant with this definition, in 2004 the Royal College of Obstetricians and Gynaecologists (RCOG) recommended that no postoperative or postdelivery patient should be left more than 6 h without voiding or catheterization (Zaki et al. 2004). In a review of compliance with these recommendations (Zaki et al. 2004), fewer than a quarter of obstetric units in England and Wales complied with the recommendation of the RCOG. With regard to the recommendations, Zaki noted that "Clear guidelines to implement strict input/output charts, measure voided volumes and check residual volume before catheterization are lacking."

In a retrospective, case-controlled study of urinary retention seen at the Mayo Clinic between August 1992 and April 2000, postpartum urinary retention after vaginal delivery occurred in 51 of 11,332 (0.45 %) of vaginal deliveries. For those women who developed urinary retention, a multivariate logistic regression identified that only instrument-assisted delivery and regional analgesia were significant independent risk factors for the condition (Carley et al. 2002).

During the first days, postpartum retention of urine is a well-known phenomenon. It can be caused by a variety of factors:

---

[1] Arbitrary in that a women might have a low bladder volume at 7 h postpartum (because of poor fluid intake), might therefore as a consequence of this low volume not have any desire to void and yet by Yip's definition might be said to be in urinary retention, even though no urologist would regard this as urinary retention.

(a) During the second stage of labor, the presenting head of the fetus presses against the urethra and the bladder and may cause edema which may act to partially obstruct flow of urine through the urethra.

(b) Lacerations and pain in the vulval region may also inhibit the voiding of urine. As well as inhibiting voiding as a consequence of causing periurethral pain, perineal trauma such as an episiotomy can cause vulval and periurethral edema, which will tend to have an obstructive effect on urine flow.

(c) The changed anatomy in the lower abdomen after birth may reduce the sensation of the bladder.

(d) Regional anesthesia (e.g., an epidural anesthetic) impairs the function of the nerves (the second, third, and fourth sacral nerves) whose function is to "drive" bladder emptying. Regional anesthesia blocks the ability of the sensory (afferent) nerves of the bladder to detect stretching of the bladder wall (bladder filling). This leads to a failure of relaxation of the muscles of the pelvic floor and the urethral sphincter mechanism and failure of contraction of the bladder. The result is the inability to void—urinary retention.

As a consequence of the above, retention of urine can occur in the postpartum period.

If unrelieved, this urinary retention can cause overdistention of the bladder. In this situation, a woman will be unable to pass urine. As the bladder becomes increasingly distended, the pressure within the bladder gradually rises. This rise in pressure subsequently causes the involuntary loss of small amounts of urine ("overflow incontinence"). In the context of epidural anesthesia, abdominal pain, which accompanies urinary retention in other circumstances, does not necessarily occur.

Bladder distention leads to temporary damage to nerve terminals within the wall of the bladder probably by reducing bladder blood supply. If bladder overdistention is maintained over several hours, then the bladder blood flow can be so much reduced that so-called ischemic damage to the sensory and motor nerve supply of the bladder can occur (the ischemia leads to the release of reactive oxygen species which mediate the nerve damage) (Ramsden et al. 1976; Brading et al. 1999).

The key to prevention of postpartum retention (and hence bladder distention injuries) is awareness of the situations in which postpartum retention occurs, ready recourse to catheterization and repeat catheterization where an initial trial of void fails, and early institution of intermittent self-catheterization (ISC) where early spontaneous voiding does not immediately return.

The Ketamine Bladder

Ketamine abuse among 16–24 year olds is on the increase from 0.8 % of individuals in that age group in 2007/2008 to 2.1 % in 2010/2011 (Smith and Flatley 2011). We have included this problem in this book because individuals with ketamine uropathy may present acutely as a urological emergency with painful hematuria (suprapubic pain), storage (irritative) LUTS, and hydronephrosis (due to a small capacity, high-pressure bladder and/or obstructive uropathy). Precisely how ketamine causes these effects remains to be established, but it or its metabolites may have a direct toxic effect on the urothe-lium, may damage the bladder's microvasculature, and may possibly cause the development of an autoimmune reaction. A vicious cycle of pain requiring the ketamine to take more ketamine for pain relief followed by more bladder damage ensues. No specific management guidelines exist as yet, but the critical thing from the perspective of the emergency urolo-gist is to be aware that a young person with hematuria and bladder pain may be abusing ketamine, and aside from the acute management of pain and hematuria, the involvement of the patient's general practitioner (GP), the chronic pain team, and drug support services is crucial to try to break the cycle of substance abuse before irreversible bladder damage occurs (Wood et al. 2011). From a pain control perspective during acute admissions, a combination of buprenorphine, co-codamol, and amitriptyline at night may help to reduce the patient's requirement for ketamine as an analgesic.

References

Abrams P, Dunn M, George N. Urodynamic findings in chronic retention of urine and their relevance to results of surgery. BMJ. 1978;2:1258–60.

Brading AF, Greenland JE, Mills IW, Symes S. Blood supply to the bladder during filling. Scand J Urol Nephrol Suppl. 1999; 201(suppl):25–31.

Carley ME, Carley JM, Vasdev G, Lesnick TG, et al. Factors that are associated with clinically overt postpartum urinary retention after vaginal delivery. Am J Obstet Gynecol. 2002;187:430–3.

Djavan B, Madersbacher S, Klingler C, Marberger M. Urodynamic assessment of patients with acute urinary retention: is treatment failure after prostatectomy predictable. J Urol. 1997;158:1829–33.

Fowler C. Urinary retention in women. Br J Urol Int. 2003;91: 463–8.

George NJR, O'Reilly PH, Barnard RJ, Blacklock NJ. High pressure chronic retention. BMJ. 1983;286:1780–3.

Hastie KJ, Dickinson AJ, Ahmad R, Moisey CU. Acute retention of urine: is trial without catheter justified? J R Coll Surg Edinb. 1990;35:225–7.

McNeill SA. Does acute urinary retention respond to alpha-blockers alone? Eur Urol. 2001;9 suppl 6:7–12.

McNeill SA, Daruwala PD, Mitchell IDC, et al. Sustained-release alfuzosin and trial without catheter after acute urinary retention. Br J Urol Int. 1999;84:622–7.

Mitchell JP. Management of chronic urinary retention. BMJ. 1984;289:515–6.

Ramsden PD, Smith JC, Dunn M, Ardran GM. Distension therapy for the unstable bladder: later results including an assessment of repeat distensions. Br J Urol. 1976;48:623–9.

Smith, K. and Flatley, J. (Eds) (2011) Drug Misuse Declared: Findings from the 2010/11 British Crime Survey. Home Office Statistical Bulletin 12/11. London: Home Office, http://www.homeoffice.gov.uk/publications/science-research-statistics/research-statistics/crime-research/hosb1211/?view=Standard&pubID=930399. Accessed on Dec. 2012.

Wood D, Cottrell A, Baker SC, et al. Recreational ketamine: from pleasure to pain. Br J Urol Int. 2011;107:1881–4.

Yip SK, Sahota D, Pang MW, Chang A. Postpartum urinary retention. Acta Scand Gynecol Scand 2004;83:881–91.

Zaki S, Pandit M, Jackson S. National survey for intrapartum and postpartum bladder care: assessing the need for guidelines. Br J Obstet Gynaecol. 2004;111:874–6.

Additional Reading

Matthias B, Schiltenwolf M. Cauda equina syndrome caused by intervertebral lumbar disc prolapse: mid-term results of 22 patients and literature review. Orthopedics. 2002;25:727–31.

Chapter 3
Nontraumatic Renal Emergencies

John Reynard

Acute Flank Pain: Ureteric or Renal Colic

Sudden onset of severe pain in the flank is most often due to the passage of a stone formed in the kidney, down through the ureter. The pain is characteristically of very sudden onset, is colicky in nature (waves of increasing severity are followed by a reduction in severity, but it seldom goes away completely), and it radiates to the groin as the stone passes into the lower ureter. The pain may change in location, from the flank to the groin, but the location of the pain does not provide a good

J. Reynard, DM, FRCS (Urol)
Department of Urology, Nuffield Department of Surgical Sciences,
Oxford University Hospitals, Oxford, UK

The National Spinal Injuries Centre, Stoke Mandeville Hospital,
Aylesbury, UK
e-mail: john.reynard@ouh.nhs.uk

H. Hashim et al. (eds.), *Urological Emergencies*
In Clinical Practice, DOI 10.1007/978-1-4471-2720-8_3,
© Springer-Verlag London 2013

indication of the position of the stone, except in those cases where the patient has pain or discomfort in the penis and a strong desire to void, which suggest that the stone may have moved into the intramural part of the ureter. The patient cannot get comfortable and may roll around in agony. Indeed, the majority of women we have seen with radiologically confirmed ureteric stones and who have also had children describe the pain of a ureteric stone as being worse than the pain of labor.

The problem with these classic symptoms of ureteric colic is that approximately 50 % of patients with the symptoms we have just described neither have a stone confirmed on subsequent imaging studies nor do they physically ever pass a stone (Smith et al. 1996; Thomson et al. 2001). They have some other cause for their pain. The list of differential diagnoses is very long. A sample of those that we have personally seen includes leaking abdominal aortic aneurysms, pneumonia, myocardial infarction, ovarian pathology (e.g., twisted ovarian cyst), acute appendicitis, testicular torsion, inflammatory bowel disease (Crohn's, ulcerative colitis), diverticulitis, ectopic pregnancy, burst peptic ulcer, bowel obstruction, renal cancers (clot colic), PUJO (pelvi-ureteric junction obstruction), and malaria (presenting as bilateral loin pain and dark hematuria—black water fever).

The point, then, in making a diagnosis is to exclude other causes of flank pain, many of which are serious and may be life-threatening (leaking aortic aneurysm, gastrointestinal causes, from those cases where the pain is due to a ureteric stone which is very rarely life-threatening).

Age of the patient can help in determining whether a diagnosis of a ureteric stone is more or less likely. Ureteric colic tends to be a disease of men (and to a lesser extent of women) between the ages of roughly 20 and 60. It does affect younger and older patients, but the range of differential diagnoses at the extremes of age, and in women, is greater. Thus, a 25-year-old man who presents with sudden onset of severe, colicky flank pain probably has a ureteric stone, but an 80-year-old woman probably has something else going on.

Distinguishing Pyelonephritis, Pyonephrosis, and Renal and Perinephric Abscess from the Simple Case of Ureteric Colic due to a Stone

These infective causes of flank pain usually present with less severe flank pain than that occurring with ureteric colic. The dominant symptoms and signs are fever, chills, nausea, and vomiting. Early differentiation between these various conditions and "simple" ureteric colic can only be made by radiological imaging.

Examination and Simple Tests

The pain from a ureteric stone is colicky in nature. It makes the patient want to move around, in an attempt to find a comfortable position. The patient may be doubled up with pain. On the other hand, patients with conditions causing peritonitis, such as appendicitis or a ruptured ectopic pregnancy, want to lie very still. Any movement is very painful, and in particular, they do not like palpation of their abdomen. Thus, when you approach patients, just spend a few seconds looking at them. If they are lying very still, you may be dealing with a non-stone cause of flank pain.

Pregnancy Test

All pre-menopausal women with acute flank pain should undergo a pregnancy test. If this is positive, they are referred to a gynecologist. If it is negative, they should undergo imaging to determine whether or not they have a ureteric stone. It goes without saying that any pre-menopausal woman who is going to undergo imaging using ionizing radiation should have a pregnancy test done first.

Dipstick or Microscopic Hematuria

While many patients with ureteric stones have dipstick or microscopic hematuria (and more rarely macroscopic hematuria), 10–30 % of such patients have no blood in their urine (Kobayashi et al. 2003; Luchs et al. 2002; Bove et al. 1999). There is evidence that if a stone has been present in the ureter for 3–4 days, there is a greater likelihood that hematuria will not be detectable.

The sensitivity of dipstick hematuria for detecting ureteric stones presenting acutely is in the order of 95 % on the first day of pain, 85 % on the second day of pain, and 65 % on the third and fourth days (Kobayashi et al. 2003). Dipstick testing is slightly more sensitive than urine microscopy for detecting stones (80 % vs. 70 %), and both ways of detecting hematuria have roughly the same specificity for diagnosing ureteric stones (about 60 %). The slightly greater sensitivity of dipstick testing over microscopy reflects the fact that seeing red blood cells depends on how good the technician is at looking for them and that they lyse and therefore disappear, if the urine specimen is not examined under the microscope within a few hours. Thus, if you see a patient with a history suggestive of ureteric colic and their pain started 3–4 days ago, they may well have no blood detectable in their urine even though they do have a stone.

The relatively poor specificity of dipstick or microscopic hematuria for detecting ureteric stones reflects the multiple other pathologies that can mimic the pain of a ureteric calculus combined with the fact that blood is detectable in a proportion of patients without demonstrable urinary tract pathology; in fact, no abnormality is found in approximately 70 % of patients with microscopic hematuria, despite full investigation with cystoscopy, renal ultrasound, and intravenous urography (IVU) (Khadra et al. 2000). Thus, blood in the urine may be a completely coincidental finding in a patient who presents with flank pain due to a non-stone cause.

Temperature

The single most important aspect of examination in patients with a ureteric stone confirmed on imaging is to measure their temperature. If patients have a stone and a fever, they may well have infection proximal to the obstructing stone. A fever in the presence of an obstructing stone is an indication for urine and blood culture, intravenous fluids and antibiotics, and nephrostomy drainage if the fever does not resolve within a matter of hours of commencement of antibiotics.

Investigation of Suspected Ureteric Colic

The intravenous urogram (IVU) was for many years the mainstay of diagnostic imaging in patients with flank pain (Fig. 3.1), and there are still some hospitals in the UK (and many in the developing world) where the IVU still forms the primary radiological investigation—hence, the continued inclusion of this test in this book. The last few years have seen a move toward computed tomography (CT) in the form of the non-contrast CT-KUB (Fig. 3.2) and where required CT urography (CTU). The CT-KUB has the following advantages over IVU:

1. It has greater specificity (95 %) and sensitivity (97 %) for diagnosing ureteric stones than has IVU (Smith et al. 1996). The CT-KUB can identify other non-stone causes of flank pain such as leaking aortic aneurysms (Fig. 3.3).
2. There is no need for contrast administration. This avoids the chance of a contrast reaction. The risk of fatal anaphylaxis following the administration of low-osmolality contrast media for IVU is on the order of 1 in 100,000 (Caro et al. 1991).

FIGURE 3.1 (a) An intravenous urogram (IVU) control film. Two calcifications are seen in the left hemipelvis. Which is the ureteric stone? (b) Following contrast administration, the lateral calcification is seen to lie outside the ureter; it is a phlebolith. The medial calcification is a ureteric stone

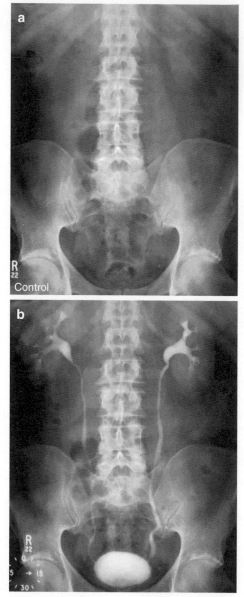

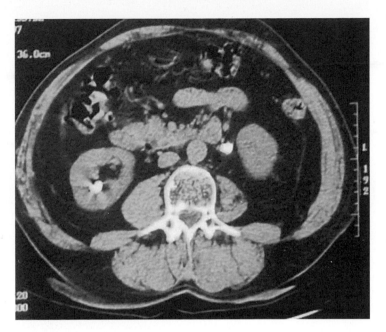

FIGURE 3.2 A computed tomography (CT) urogram (CTU). Stones "light" up as very radiodense structures. There is one in the left ureter and one in the right kidney

3. A CT-KUB is faster, taking just a few minutes to image the kidneys and ureters. An IVU, particularly where delayed films are required to identify a stone causing high-grade obstruction, may take hours to identify the precise location of the obstructing stone (Fig. 3.4).

4. In some hospitals, where high volumes of CT scans are done, the cost of a CT-KUB is equivalent to that of IVU (Thomson et al. 2001).

If you only have access to IVU, remember that it is contraindicated in patients with a history of previous contrast reactions and should be avoided in those with hay fever or a strong history of allergies or asthma who have not been pre-treated with high-dose steroids 24 h before the IVU. Patients taking metformin for diabetes should stop this for 48 h prior

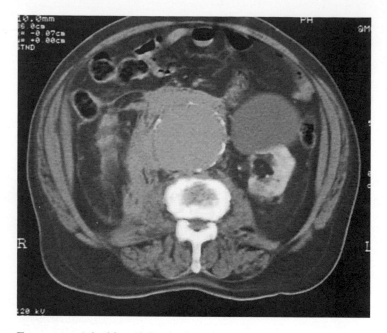

FIGURE 3.3 A leaking abdominal aortic aneurysm, referred as a ureteric stone, but correctly diagnosed by CTU

to an IVU. Clearly, being able to perform an alternative test in such patients, such as a CT-KUB, is very useful.

In hospitals where 24-h access to the CT-KUB is not possible, patients with suspected ureteric colic may be admitted for pain relief and undergo a CT-KUB the following morning. It is our policy, when a CT-KUB is not immediately available (between the hours of midnight and 8 a.m.), to perform an abdominal ultrasound in all patients over the age of 50 years who present with flank pain suggestive of a possible stone. This is done to exclude serious pathology such as a leaking abdominal aortic aneurysm and to demonstrate any other gross abnormalities due to non-stone-associated flank pain.

Plain abdominal x-ray and renal ultrasound are not sufficiently sensitive or specific for their routine use for diagnosing stones.

FIGURE 3.4 (**a**) On a 1-h postcontrast film, the right ureter is still not opacified. Only the outline of the kidney and renal collecting system is visible because of the distal obstruction. (**b**) In this case, it takes 2 h for the IVU to demonstrate the stone and its position in the right lower ureter

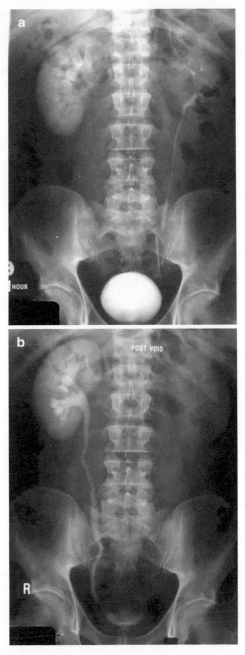

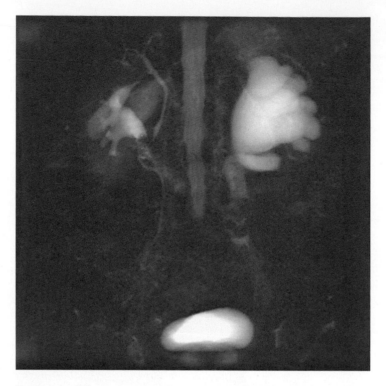

FIGURE 3.5 Magnetic resonance urogram. Stones appear as "black holes"

Magnetic Resonance Urography (Fig. 3.5)

This is said to be an accurate way of determining whether or not a stone is present in the ureter (Louca et al. 1999; O'Malley et al. 1997).

However, at the present time, cost, restricted availability, and the difficulty (in our experience) that radiologists often seem to have in interpreting an investigation they very seldom carry out limit its usefulness as a routine diagnostic method of imaging in cases of acute flank pain. This may change as MR scanners become more widely available, but in the 7 years since the first edition of this book we have seen no increase in the use of MRU — CT-KUB remains the investigation of choice.

Acute Management of Ureteric Stones

The management of any acutely presenting ureteric stone starts with pain control and NSAIDs such as diclofenac (Voltarol) given by intramuscular or intravenous injection, by mouth, or per rectum can, in many cases, provide rapid and effective pain control (Laerum et al. 1996). In other cases, opiate analgesics such as pethidine or morphine are required, in addition to NSAIDs. Desmopressin (DDAVP) as a nasal spray (40 μg) can reduce the pain of ureteric colic presumably by reducing intrarenal pressure and possibly by a direct action in reducing ureteric contraction (Leslie 2001). The antiemetic metoclopramide (10 mg iv) provides rapid relief from nausea.

There is no need to encourage the patient to drink copious amounts of fluids or to give them large volumes of fluids intravenously, in the hope that this will "flush" the stone out. A randomized trial of forced intravenous hydration compared to minimal hydration showed no significant difference in analgesic requirement, pain scores, or spontaneous stone passage rates (Springhart et al. 2006).

Renal blood flow and urine output from the affected kidney will tend to fall during an episode of acute partial obstruction due to a stone, and any excess fluid that is excreted will tend to cause a greater degree of hydronephrosis in the affected kidney, which will make ureteric peristalsis even less efficient than it already is. Remember, peristalsis, the forward propulsion of a bolus of urine down the ureter, can occur only if the walls of the ureter above the bolus of urine can coapt, that is, close firmly together. If they cannot, as occurs in a ureter distended with urine, the bolus of urine cannot move distally. This is why insertion of a percutaneous nephrostomy tube can restore efficient peristalsis. By draining the hydronephrosis and hydroureter, it allows the ureteric wall to coapt and thus encourages a return to normal peristaltic function.

Medical Expulsive Therapy for Stones (MET)

There is a growing body of evidence supporting the efficacy of MET with the smooth muscle-relaxing alpha-1 adrenergic adrenoceptor blockers, such as tamsulosin. The evidence suggests that they probably increase spontaneous stone passage rates, reduce stone passage time, and reduce the frequency of episodes of ureteric colic (Dellabella 2003; Parsons et al. 2007). The EAU/AUA Nephrolithiasis Guideline Panel meta-analysis showed that 29 % more patients (CI: 20–37 %) taking tamsulosin passed their stones compared with controls (Preminger 2007). Tamsulosin has been most studied in this setting, but other alpha-blockers appear to be equally effective (Zehri et al. 2010; Agrawal et al. 2009; Yilmaz et al. 2005). Whether stones in all segments of the ureter are equally responsive to alpha-blockers remains to be determined.

Zhu's meta-analysis (Zhu 2009) of seven studies comprising 484 patients suggests that 0.4 mg of tamsulosin also seems to encourage stone clearance after ESWL for ureteric (and possibly renal) stones (pooled absolute risk difference in spontaneous stone passage 19 % in favor of tamsulosin—if 70 % pass their stones spontaneously without tamsulosin, 89 % pass their stones with tamsulosin). Five patients needed to be treated with tamsulosin to achieve stone clearance in one, and the mean difference in time to stone expulsion was 8 days in favor of those on tamsulosin.

In a study of 1,596 patients with distal ureteric stones (size range 4–7 mm) randomized to tamsulosin and 1,593 to the calcium channel blocker nifedipine and using a 4-week follow-up CT scan to determine if the stone had passed, time to stone expulsion in the tamsulosin group was 78 h compared to 138 h in the nifedipine group (Zhangqun et al. 2010). Glyceryl trinitrate patches do not increase stone passage or reduce frequency of pain episodes, and corticosteroids are of minimal, if any, benefit (Hussain 2001).

Indications for Intervention to Relieve Obstruction and/or Remove the Stone

1. Pain that fails to respond to analgesics, or that initially does so but then recurs and cannot be controlled with additional pain relief, is an indication for drainage of the kidney (by JJ stent insertion or percutaneous nephrostomy) or emergency definitive treatment of the stone.
2. Where there is an associated fever, one should have a low threshold for draining the kidney, and this is usually done by percutaneous nephrostomy.
3. Where renal function is impaired because of the stone (solitary kidney obstructed by a stone, bilateral ureteric stones, or preexisting renal impairment that gets worse as a consequence of a ureteric stone), the threshold for intervention is lower.
4. Obstruction unrelieved for >4 weeks can result in long-term loss of renal function. In a study of 239 patients presenting with unilateral ureteric stones, after 2 weeks the stones were still present in 143 patients (Holm-Nielsen et al. 1981). Of these 143 patients, 50% had renal obstruction defined by isotope renography; 11 of 31 patients (35 %) with obstruction for >4 weeks developed varying degrees of irreversible renal damage. The problem with current imaging for stones, which nowadays is essentially CTU, is the absence of any information on the presence of renal obstruction (most urologists do not routinely obtain isotope renograms in patients with ureteric colic). However, what we do know from the Holm-Nielsen study is that only 50 % of patients with ureteric stones that are still present at 2 weeks have renographic evidence of obstruction. It seems reasonable to limit the period of watchful waiting for spontaneous stone passage to approximately 4 weeks and to intervene to remove the stone or drain the kidney (e.g., by JJ stent placement) if it has not passed at this time.

5. Personal or occupational reasons. As stated above, some
patients will not be able to wait for spontaneous stone passage and therefore may accept the risks associated with
active intervention. The classic example would be the air-
line pilot who is unable to fly until he is stone-free.

Emergency Temporizing and Definitive Treatment of the Stone

Where the pain of a ureteric stone fails to respond to analgesics
or where renal function is impaired because of the stone, then
temporary relief of the obstruction can be obtained by insertion of a JJ stent or percutaneous nephrostomy tube. This has
the advantage of not taking much time to perform. However,
the disadvantage is that the stone is still present. While the
stone may pass down and out of the ureter with a stent in situ,
in many instances the stone simply sits where it is, and subsequent definitive treatment is still required. Furthermore, though
a JJ stent can relieve the pain due to the stone, it can cause
bothersome storage (irritative) bladder symptoms (pain in the
bladder, frequency, and urgency). Having said this, a JJ stent
will usually result in passive dilatation of the ureter so that
subsequent stone treatment in the form of ureteroscopy is technically easier and therefore more likely to be successful.
Similarly, by allowing passive dilatation of the ureter, fragments
of stone produced by extracorporeal shock wave lithotripsy
(ESWL) may be more easily able to pass out of the ureter.

General options for definitive treatment of a ureteric
stone are ESWL and ureteroscopic stone removal. ESWL is
suitable for stones in the upper and lower ureter. Ureteroscopy
can be used to treat stones at any level in the ureter, although
access and fragmentation of stones in the lower ureter is generally easier (Fig. 3.6).

Whether you decide to carry out definitive stone treatment, and what type of treatment you offer, will depend
on local facilities and expertise. Many hospitals do not
have daily access to ESWL. In others, surgeons with
experience of ureteroscopic stone fragmentation are not
always available.

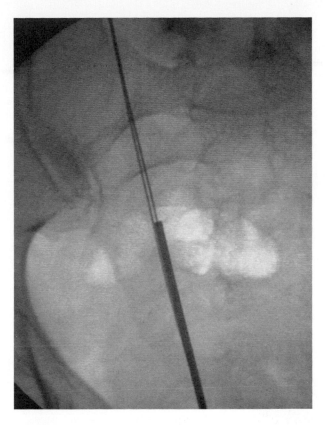

FIGURE 3.6 Ureteroscopic approach to a lower ureteric stone. Note the presence of two guidewires—one is a "safety" line; the ureteroscope is passed over the other to the level of the stone

Emergency Treatment of an Obstructed, Infected Kidney

The rationale for performing percutaneous nephrostomy (Fig. 3.7) rather than JJ stent insertion (Fig. 3.8) for an infected, obstructed kidney is to reduce the likelihood of septicemia occurring as a consequence of showering bacteria into the circulation. In reality, there is no difference in outcome in those patients with infected, obstructed kidneys who are stented compared with those whose obstruction is

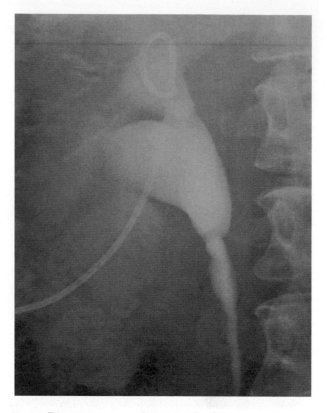

FIGURE 3.7 Percutaneous nephrostomy in situ

relieved by nephrostomy drainage (Pearle 1998). The EAU/
AUA Nephrolithiasis Guideline Panel (Preminger 2007) rec-
ommends that the system of drainage (whether JJ stent or
nephrostomy) should be left to the discretion of the urologist.
This recommendation is based on a randomized trial in which
JJ stent insertion and nephrostomy were shown to be equally
effective in terms of time to normalization of temperature
and white count (which takes approximately 2–3 days) and in
hospital stay in a group of 42 patients with obstructing stones
and a temperature of >38 °C and/or white blood count of
17,000/mm^3. A 6- or 7-Ch JJ stent (with a Foley bladder

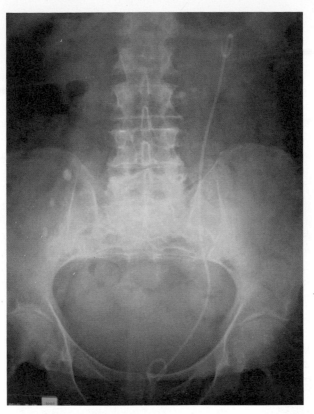

FIGURE 3.8 JJ stent post-insertion

catheter in 70 %) or 8-Ch (occasionally larger) nephrostomy (plus a urethral catheter in 33 %) was used.

Other Non-stone Causes of Acute Flank Pain

These include pelvi-ureteric junction obstruction (PUJO), which is called ureteropelvic junction obstruction (UPJO) in North America, and infective causes such as acute pyelonephritis, emphysematous pyelonephritis, and xanthogranulomatous pyelonephritis.

Pelvi-Ureteric Junction Obstruction

This is a functional impairment of transport of urine from the renal pelvis into the ureter. It may be acquired or congenital. The majority of cases are probably congenital in origin, but do not always present in childhood. Indeed, many present in young adults. The precise cause of the aperistaltic segment of ureter that leads to congenital cases of this condition is not known. Acquired causes of PUJO include stones (the investigation and management of which is discussed above), urothelial tumors (transitional cell carcinoma), and inflammatory and postoperative strictures.

Not infrequently PUJO may present acutely with flank pain, which may be severe enough to mimic a ureteric stone. When imaging (nowadays usually a CT scan) demonstrates hydronephrosis, with a normal-caliber ureter below the pelvi-ureteric junction (PUJ) and no stone (or tumor) is seen, the diagnosis of PUJO becomes likely, and a renogram (e.g., MAG3 scan) should be done to confirm the diagnosis (Fig. 3.9).

Acute Pyelonephritis

Clinical Definition

This is infective inflammation of the kidney and renal pelvis, but more usefully from a clinical perspective, the diagnosis is a clinical one, that is, based on the symptoms and signs of fever, flank pain, and tenderness, often with an elevated white count. It may affect one or both kidneys. There are usually—but not always—accompanying symptoms suggestive of a lower urinary tract infection (frequency, urgency, suprapubic

---

FIGURE 3.9 (**a**) Right pelvi-ureteric junction (PUJ) obstruction on ultrasound. (**b**) PUJ obstruction on CT. Note the normal-caliber ureter with hydronephrosis above. (**c**) MAG3 renogram of PUJ obstruction demonstrating obstruction to excretion of radioisotope by the kidney (See this figure in full color in the insert)

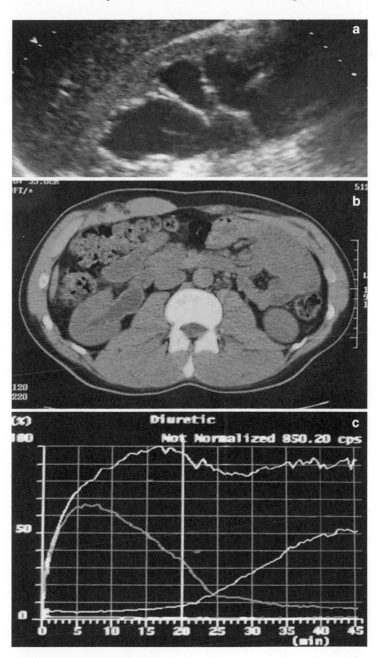

pain, urethral burning, or pain on voiding) that led to the ascending infection, which resulted in the subsequent acute pyelonephritis. The infecting organisms are commonly *Escherichia coli* (80 % of cases), Enterococci (*Streptococcus faecalis*), *Klebsiella*, *Proteus*, and *Pseudomonas*.

Urine culture is positive for bacterial growth, but in 20 % of patients, the bacterial count may be <100,000 colony-forming units (cfu)/mL of urine (Rubin et al. 1992)—the strict definition for urinary infection. Thus, if you suspect a diagnosis of acute pyelonephritis from the symptoms of fever and flank pain, but there are only 1,000 cfu/mL, manage the case as acute pyelonephritis.

Investigation and Treatment

Acute pyelonephritis may be categorized as (1) uncomplicated—not warranting hospital admission, (2) uncomplicated—warranting hospital admission for intravenous antibiotics, but with normal urinary tracts, and (3) complicated—those with catheters or other urinary tract abnormalities (e.g., renal obstruction due to a ureteric stone).

For those patients who have a fever but are not systemically unwell (group 1), outpatient management is reasonable. Culture the urine and start oral antibiotics according to your local antibiotic policy (which will be based on the likely infecting organisms and their likely antibiotic sensitivity). We use oral ciprofloxacin, 500 mg twice daily for 10 days.

If the patient is systemically unwell (groups 2 and 3), admit them to hospital, culture urine and blood, and start intravenous fluids and intravenous antibiotics, again selecting the antibiotic according to your local antibiotic policy. We use IV ampicillin 1 g three times a day and gentamicin, 5 mg/kg as a once daily dose.

Distinguishing between groups 2 and 3—both being unwell enough to require hospitalization, but with one having an abnormal urinary tract and the other not—is based on radiological imaging (unless the patient can tell you they have an underlying urinary tract abnormality).

When Should Radiological Imaging Be Done

The American College of Radiology Appropriateness Criteria for imaging in cases of acute pyelonephritis (last updated 2008) state that kidney ultrasound scanning:

> adds little to management if the patient responds to therapy within 72 hours...patients with uncomplicated pyelonephritis probably need no radiologic workup if they respond to antibiotic therapy within 72 hours. If there is no response to therapy CT of the abdomen and pelvis is the study of choice. Diabetics or other immunocompromised patients should probably be evaluated with pre-contrast and post-contrast CT within 24 hours of diagnosis, if response is not prompt. Ultrasound should be reserved for patients in whom pyonephrosis is suspected and those patients for whom exposure to contrast or radiation is hazardous.
> www.acr.org/secondarymainmenucategories/quality_safety/app_criteria/pdf/expertpanelonurologicimaging/acutepyelonephritis-doc3.aspx

The European Association of Urology Guidelines (Grabe et al. 2012, *Guidelines on Urological Infections*, page 16—Updated March 2011) state that:

> Evaluation of the upper urinary tract with ultrasound should be performed to rule out urinary obstruction or renal stone disease. Additional investigations, such as an unenhanced helical computed tomography (CT), [*or*] excretory urography...should be considered if the patients remain febrile after 72 h of treatment. The CT appearances of a typical case of acute pyelonephritis is shown in (Fig. 3.10).

In our opinion, these guidelines need to be interpreted with caution. It can be difficult on clinical grounds to distinguish a patient with an uncomplicated pyelonephritis from one with one of the more serious conditions that mimic pyelonephritis such as pyonephrosis, an obstructed ureteric stone with infection within the obstructed collecting system, or emphysematous pyelonephritis. We tend to arrange a KUB x-ray and ultrasound within 24 h of admission in all cases that we feel warrant hospitalization. Where there is hydronephrosis or a suggestion on the x-ray of a stone, a CT-KUB should be done to determine if there is an obstructing lesion such as a ureteric stone. Most ultrasound scans are

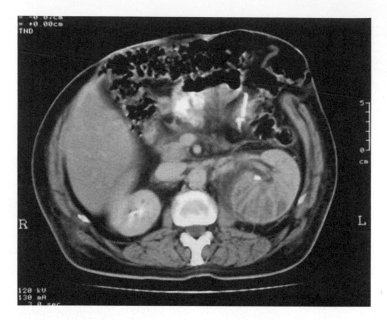

FIGURE 3.10 A CTU without contrast in a diabetic patient with left acute pyelonephritis. Note the incidental finding of a nonobstructing left renal calculus

normal, but it is always a relief to diagnose an obstructed, infected system earlier rather than later.

Where the guidelines are strictly applied, the lack of response to treatment indicates that you are dealing with a pyonephrosis (i.e., pus in the kidney, which like any abscess will respond only to drainage), a perinephric abscess (which again will respond only to drainage), or emphysematous pyelonephritis. The CTU may demonstrate an obstructing ureteric calculus that may have been missed on the KUB x-ray and ultrasound and will show a perinephric abscess if present. The problem with waiting 72 h to determine if this is a patient who has failed to respond (and arranging imaging only once this failure to respond becomes apparent) is that by this time, you may have a very sick patient on your hands in whom "the boat has been missed." Some such patients may not be recoverable.

If the patient responds to IV antibiotics, change to an oral antibiotic of appropriate sensitivity when they become apyrexial and continue this for approximately 10–14 days.

Infected Hydronephrosis and Pyonephrosis

Infected hydronephrosis is bacterial infection in a hydronephrotic kidney. Pyonephrosis is an infected hydronephrosis with destruction of renal parenchyma and pus formation, the infection being severe enough to cause accumulation of pus within the renal pelvis and calyces of the kidney and if allowed to run its course, leading to complete loss of renal function. Clinically it is difficult to distinguish the two. The causes are essentially those of hydronephrosis, where infection has supervened. Thus, they include ureteric obstruction by stone and PUJ obstruction.

Patients with pyonephrosis are usually very unwell, with a high fever, flank pain, and tenderness. Again, a patient with this combination of symptoms and signs will usually be investigated by a renal ultrasound (which will show a hydronephrosis—Fig. 3.11) followed by a renal CT.

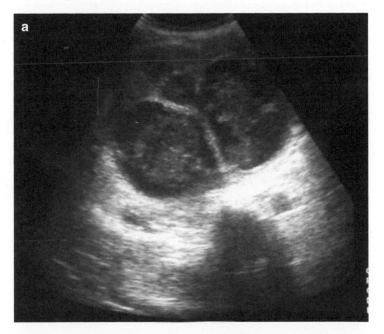

FIGURE 3.11 (a) The appearance of a pyonephrosis on ultrasound. Note the hyperreflective material within the dilated system. (b) A right pyonephrosis on CT, done without contrast. Note the presence of a stone in the kidney. (c) A right pyonephrosis on CT postcontrast administration

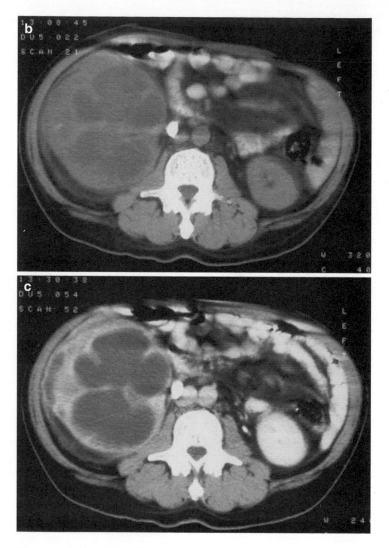

FIGURE 3.11 (continued)

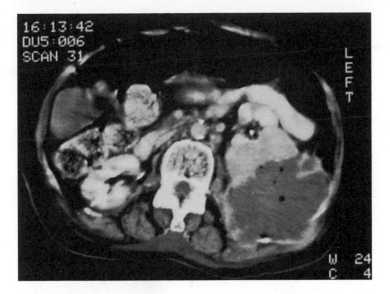

FIGURE 3.12 A left perinephric abscess as seen on CT

Treatment consists of IV antibiotics (as for pyelonephritis), IV fluids, and percutaneous nephrostomy insertion.

Perinephric Abscess

Perinephric abscess (Fig. 3.12) develops as a consequence of extension of infection outside the parenchyma of the kidney in acute pyelonephritis (a cortical abscess ruptures into the surrounding perirenal tissues), or more rarely, nowadays, from hematogenous spread of infection from a distant site. The abscess develops within Gerota's fascia — the fascial layer surrounding the kidneys and their cushion of perinephric fat (rupture through Gerota's fascia creates a "paranephric" abscess, but infections of the bowel, pancreas, and pleural space may also cause development of a paranephric abscess as an extension of a vertebral osteomyelitis). *E. coli*, *Proteus*, and *S. aureus* are the common infecting organisms.

One-third of patients are diabetic, and associated conditions such as an obstructing ureteric calculus may be the precipitating event leading to development of the perinephric abscess. Failure of a seemingly straightforward case of acute pyelonephritis to respond to intravenous antibiotics within a few days should arouse your suspicion that there is something else going on, such as the accumulation of pus in or around the kidney or obstruction with infection. Imaging studies, such as ultrasound and more especially CT, will establish the diagnosis (clearly, the sooner they are done, the earlier will it be possible to distinguish between the straightforward case of pyelonephritis and that of a perinephric abscess). Radiographically controlled percutaneous drainage of the abscess with intravenous antibiotic therapy is the mainstays of management. However, if the pus collection is large, formal open surgical drainage under general anesthetic will provide more effective drainage.

Emphysematous Pyelonephritis

This is a rare and severe form of acute, necrotizing infection of the renal parenchyma and perirenal tissues caused by gas-forming organisms (Fig. 3.13). It is characterized by fever and abdominal pain, with radiographic evidence of gas within and around the kidney (on plain radiography or CT). It usually occurs in diabetics (though not exclusively so) and, in many cases, is precipitated by urinary obstruction by, for example, ureteric stones. The high glucose levels of the poorly controlled diabetic provide an ideal environment for fermentation by enterobacteria, carbon dioxide being produced during this process.

Presentation

Emphysematous pyelonephritis presents as a severe acute pyelonephritis (high fever and systemic upset) that fails to respond within 2–3 days with conventional treatment in the

form of intravenous antibiotics. *E. coli* is a common causative organism, with *Klebsiella* and *Proteus* occurring from
time to time. Obtaining a KUB x-ray and ultrasound in all
patients with acute pyelonephritis may allow earlier diagnosis of this rare form of pyelonephritis. An unusual distribu-
tion of gas on x-ray may suggest that the gas lies around the
kidney (e.g., crescent or kidney shaped). Renal ultrasonogra
phy often demonstrates strong focal echoes, due to the

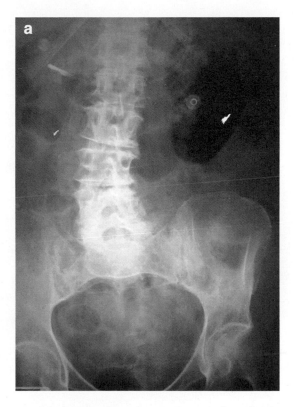

FIGURE 3.13 **(a)** A case of emphysematous pyelonephritis on plain
abdominal x-ray. Note the presence of gas within the left kidney.
(b) A CT of the same case. The gas in the kidney (like that in the
bowel) is black on CT. **(c)** A percutaneous drain has been inserted with
the patient lying prone. Note the J loop of the drain in the kidney

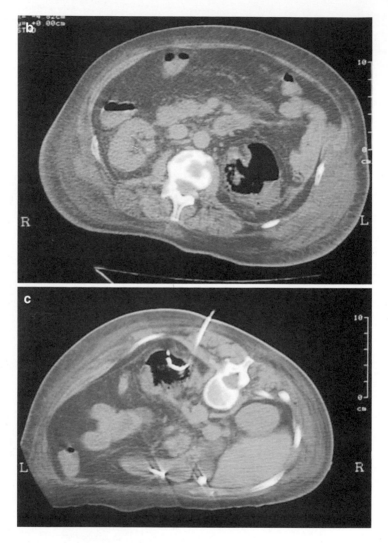

FIGURE 3.13 (continued)

presence of gas within the kidney. Intrarenal gas will be clearly seen on CT scan.

Treatment

Patients with emphysematous pyelonephritis are usually very unwell. Mortality is high. The initial approach in all patients has evolved over from an aggressive surgical approach to a conservative one with intravenous antibiotics and fluids, percutaneous drainage, and careful control of diabetes. Between 66 and 92 % of patients managed in this way will not need to progress to nephrectomy (Aswathaman et al. 2008). In those where sepsis is poorly controlled, reimaging may identify further pockets of infection which can be drained percutaneously, and as many as one-third of patients may require additional drainage (Aswathaman et al. 2008). Nephrectomy is required.

Acute Pyelonephritis, Pyonephrosis, Perinephric Abscess, and Emphysematous Pyelonephritis: Making the Diagnosis

Maintaining a degree of suspicion in all cases of presumed acute pyelonephritis is the single most important thing in making an early diagnosis of complicated renal infection, such as a pyonephrosis, perinephric abscess, or emphysematous pyelonephritis. If patients are very unwell or diabetic or have a history suggestive of stones, for example, ask yourself whether they may have something more than just a simple acute pyelonephritis. They may give a history of sudden onset of severe flank pain a few days earlier, which suggests that they may have passed a stone into their ureter at this stage and that later infection supervened.

A policy of arranging for a KUB x-ray and renal ultrasound in all patients with suspected renal infection is wise.

The main clinical indicators that suggest you may be dealing with a more complex form of renal infection are length of symptoms prior to treatment and time taken to respond to treatment. Thorley and colleagues (1974) reviewed a series of 52 patients with perinephric abscess. They noted that the majority of patients with uncomplicated acute pyelonephritis had been symptomatic for less than 5 days, whereas most of those with a perinephric abscess had been symptomatic for more than 5 days prior to hospitalization. In addition, all patients with acute pyelonephritis became afebrile after 4 days of treatment with an appropriate antibiotic, whereas patients with perinephric abscesses remained pyrexial.

Xanthogranulomatous Pyelonephritis

This is a severe renal infection usually (though not always) occurring in association with underlying renal calculi (about 80 % of patients have stones—approximately half of these being staghorn calculi) and renal obstruction. The severe infection results in destruction of renal tissue, and a nonfunctioning, enlarged kidney is the end result.

E. coli and *Proteus* are common causative organisms. Macrophages full of fat become deposited around abscesses within the parenchyma of the kidney (so-called lipid-laden foamy macrophages, which are difficult to distinguish from clear cell renal carcinoma on frozen section biopsies). The infection may be confined to the kidney or extend to the perinephric fat. The kidney becomes grossly enlarged, though with a normal contour and macroscopically contains yellowish nodules, pus, and areas of hemorrhagic necrosis. It can be very difficult to distinguish the radiological findings from a renal cancer on imaging studies such as CT (Fig. 3.14). Indeed, in most cases, the diagnosis is made after nephrectomy for a presumed renal cell carcinoma.

Presentation and Imaging Studies

Patients present acutely with flank pain and fever, with a tender flank mass. Bacteria (*E. coli*, *Proteus*) may be found on urine culture. Renal ultrasonography shows an enlarged

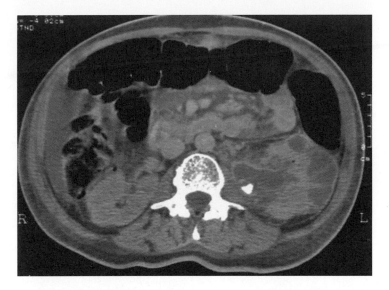

FIGURE 3.14 A case of xanthogranulomatous pyelonephritis (*left*) as seen on CT. This can be very difficult to distinguish radiologically from a renal cancer

kidney containing echogenic material. On CT, renal calcification is usually seen, within the renal mass. Non-enhancing cavities are seen, containing pus and debris. On radioisotope scanning, there is usually little or no function in the affected kidney.

Management

On presentation, these patients are usually commenced on antibiotics as the constellation of symptoms and signs suggest infection. When imaging studies are done, such as CT, the appearances usually suggest the possibility of a renal cell carcinoma, and therefore, when signs of infection have resolved, the majority of patients will proceed to nephrectomy. Only following pathological examination of the removed kidney will it become apparent that the diagnosis was one of infection (xanthogranulomatous pyelonephritis) rather than one of a tumor.

References

Agrawal M, Gupta M, Gupta A, et al. Prospective randomized trial comparing efficacy of alfuzosin and tamsulosin in management of lower ureteral stones. Urology. 2009;73:706–9.

Aswathaman K, Gopalakrishnan G, Gnanaraj L, et al. Emphysematous pyelonephritis: outcome of conservative management. Urology. 2008;71:1007–9.

Bove P, Kaplan D, Dalrymple N, et al. Re-examining the value of hematuria testing in patients with acute flank pain. J Urol. 1999;162:685–7.

Caro JJ, Trindale E, McGregor M. The risks of death and severe non-fatal reactions with high vs. low osmolality contrast media. AJR. 1991;156:825–32.

Dellabella M. Efficacy of tamsulosin in the medical management of juxtavesicalureteral stones. J Urol. 2003;170:2202–5.

Grabe M, Bjerklund-Johansen TE, Botto H, Wullt B, Çek M, Naber KG, Pickard RS, Tenke P, Wagenlehner F. The European Association of urology guidelines on urological infections. Arnhem: European Association of Urology; 2012. p. 16.

Holm-Nielsen A, Jorgensen T, Mogensen P, Fogh J. The prognostic value of probe renography in ureteric stone obstruction. Br J Urol. 1981;53:504–7.

Hussain Z. Use of glyceryl trinitrate patches in patients with ureteral stones: a randomized, double-blind, placebo-controlled study. Urology. 2001;58:521–5.

Khadra MH, Pickard RS, Charlton M, et al. A prospective analysis of 1,930 patients with hematuria to evaluate current diagnostic practice. J Urol. 2000;163:524–7.

Kobayashi T, Nishizawa K, Mitsumori K, Ogura K. Impact of date of onset on the absence of hematuria in patients with acute renal colic. J Urol. 2003;1770:1093–6.

Laerum E, Ommundsen OE, Granseth J, et al. Intramuscular diclofenac versus intravenous indomethacin in the treatment of acute renal colic. Eur Urol. 1996;30:358–62.

Leslie SW. An assessment of the clinical efficacy of intranasal desmopressin spray in the treatment of renal colic. BJU Int. 2001;87:322–5.

Louca G, Liberopoulos K, Fidas A, et al. MR urography in the diagnosis of urinary tract obstruction. Eur Urol. 1999;35:14.

Luchs JS, Katz DS, Lane DS, et al. Utility of hematuria testing in patients with suspected renal colic: correlation with unenhanced helical CT results. Urology. 2002;59:839.

O'Malley ME, Soto JA, Yucel EK, Hussain S. MR urography: evaluation of a three-dimensional fast spin-echo technique in patients with hydronephrosis. AJR. 1997;168:387–92.

Parsons JK, Hergan LA, Sakamoto K, et al. Efficacy of alpha blockers for the treatment of ureteral stones. J Urol. 2007;177:983–7.

Pearle MS. Optimal method of urgent decompression of the collecting system for obstruction and infection due to ureteral calculi. J Urol. 1998;160:1260.

Preminger GM. 2007 Guideline for the management of ureteral calculi Joint EAU/AUA Nephrolithiasis Guideline Panel. J Urol. 2007;178:2418–34.

Rubin RH, Shapiro ED, Andriole VT, Davis RJ, Stamm WE. Evaluation of new anti-infective drugs for the treatment of urinary tract infection. Infectious Diseases Society of America and the Food and Drug Administration. Clin Infect Dis. 1992;15 Suppl 1:S216–7.

Smith RC, Verga M, McCarthy S, Rosenfield AT. Diagnosis of acute flank pain: value of unenhanced helical CT. AJR. 1996; 166:97–101.

Springhart WP, Marguet CG, Sur RL, et al. Forced versus minimal intravenous hydration in the management of acute renal colic: a randomized trial. J Endourol. 2006;20:713–6.

Thomson JM, Glocer J, Abbott C, et al. Computed tomography versus intravenous urography in diagnosis of acute flank pain from urolithiasis: a randomized study comparing imaging costs and radiation dose. Australas Radiol. 2001;45:291–7.

Thorley JD, Jones SR, Sanford JP. Perinephric abscess. Medicine. 1974;58:441.

Yilmaz E, Batislam E, Basar MM, et al. The comparison and efficacy of 3 different alpha 1 adrenergic blockers for distal ureteric stones. J Urol. 2005;173:2010.

Zehri AA, Ather MH, Abbas F, Biyabani SR. Preliminary study of efficacy of doxazosin as a medical expulsive therapy of distal ureteric stones in a randomized clinical trial. Urology. 2010;75:1285–8.

Zhangqun Y, Huan Y, Hong L, et al. A multicentre, prospective, randomized trial: comparative efficacy of tamsulosin and nifedipine in medical expulsive therapy for distal ureteric stones with renal colic. Br J Urol Int. 2010;108:276–9.

Zhu Y. Alpha blockers to assist stone clearance after extra-corporeal shock wave lithotripsy: a meta-analysis. BJU Int. 2009;106:256–61.

Chapter 4
Other Infective Urological Emergencies

Hashim Hashim

Urinary Septicemia

Sepsis as a result of a urinary tract infection is a serious condition that can lead to septic shock and death. Septicemia or sepsis is the clinical syndrome caused by bacterial infection of the blood, confirmed by positive blood cultures for a specific organism. There should be a documented source of infection with a systemic response to the infection. The systemic response is known as the systemic inflammatory response syndrome (SIRS) and is defined as at least two of the following:

- Fever (>38 °C) or hypothermia (<36 °C)
- Tachycardia (>90 bpm, in patients not on beta-blockers)
- Tachypnea (respiratory rate >20 breaths/min or $PaCO_2 < 4.3$ kPa (<32 mmHg) or a requirement for mechanical ventilation)
- White cell count >12,000 cells/mm^3, <4,000 cells/mm^3, or 10% immature (band) forms

Severe sepsis or sepsis syndrome is a state of altered organ perfusion or evidence of dysfunction of one or more organs, with at least one of the following: hypoxemia, lactic acidosis, oliguria, or altered mental status.

H. Hashim, M.D., FEBU, FRCS (Urol)
Consultant Urological Surgeon and Director of the Urodynamics Unit,
Department of Urology, Bristol Urological Institute,
Southmead Hospital, Bristol, UK
e-mail: h.hashim@gmail.com

H. Hashim et al. (eds.), *Urological Emergencies*
In Clinical Practice, DOI 10.1007/978-1-4471-2720-8_4,
© Springer-Verlag London 2013

Septic shock is severe sepsis with refractory hypotension, hypoperfusion, and organ dysfunction. This is a life-threatening condition.

There are many causes of urinary sepsis, but in the hospital setting, the commonest causes from a urological perspective are the presence of or manipulation of indwelling urinary catheters, urinary tract surgery, particularly endoscopic transurethral resection of the prostate (TURP), transurethral resection of bladder tumor (TURBT), ureteroscopy, percutaneous nephrolithotomy (PCNL), and urinary tract obstruction, particularly that due to stones obstructing the ureter. In the National Prostatectomy Audit and the European Collaborative Study of Antibiotic Prophylaxis for TURP, septicemia occurred in approximately 1.5% of men undergoing TURP. Diabetic patients, patients in the intensive care units (ICU), and patients on chemotherapy and steroids are more prone to urosepsis.

The commonest causative organisms of urinary sepsis are *Escherichia coli*, enterococci (*Streptococcus faecalis*), staphylococci, *Pseudomonas aeruginosa*, *Klebsiella*, and *Proteus mirabilis*.

The principles of management include early recognition, resuscitation, localization of the source of sepsis, early and appropriate antibiotic administration, and removal of the primary source of sepsis. The clinical scenario is usually a postoperative patient who has undergone TURP or surgery for stones. Having returned to the ward, the patient becomes pyrexial, starts to shiver and shake, is tachycardic, and may be confused. On inspection, the patient may initially show signs of peripheral vasodilatation (may appear flushed and warm to the touch). Look for symptoms and signs of a non-urological source of sepsis such as pneumonia. If there are no indications of infection elsewhere, assume the urinary tract is the source of sepsis.

Investigations

- Urine culture. An immediate gram stain may aid in deciding which antibiotic to use.

- Full blood count. The white blood count is usually elevated. The platelet count may be low, a possible indication of impending disseminated intravascular coagulopathy (DIC).
- Coagulation screen. This is important if surgical or radiological drainage of the source of infection is necessary.
- Urea and electrolytes as a baseline determination of renal function.
- Arterial blood gases to identify hypoxia and the presence of metabolic acidosis.
- Blood cultures.
- Chest X-ray (CXR), looking for pneumonia, atelectasis, and effusions.

Depending on the clinical situation, a renal ultrasound may be helpful to demonstrate hydronephrosis or pyonephrosis and CT urography (CTU) may be used to establish the presence or absence of a ureteric stone (non-contrast CT being the most important phase of the CTU, to look for stones).

Treatment

- Remember A (airway), B (breathing), C (circulation).
- Administer 100% oxygen via a face mask.
- Establish intravenous access with a wide-bore intravenous cannula, e.g., 16G or 18G.
- Start an intravenous infusion of crystalloid, e.g., normal saline or colloid, e.g., Gelofusin.
- Catheterize the patient to monitor urine output.
- Start empirical antibiotic therapy (see below). This should be adjusted later when cultures are available.
- If there is septic shock, the patient needs to be transferred to the intensive care unit (ICU). Inotropic support may be needed. Steroids may be used as adjunctive therapy in gram-negative infections. Naloxone may help revert endotoxic shock. This should all be done under the supervision of an intensivist.

- Treat the underlying cause. Drain any obstruction and remove any foreign body. If there is a stone obstructing the ureter, then either ask the radiologist to insert a nephrostomy tube to relieve the obstruction or take the patient to the operating room and insert a JJ stent. Send any urine specimens obtained for microscopy and culture.

Empirical Treatment

Empirical antibiotic treatment is the "blind" use of antibiotics based on an educated guess of the most likely pathogen that has caused the sepsis. In urinary sepsis, the cause is often a gram-negative rod. Gram-negative aerobic rods include the enterobacteria, e.g., *E. coli*, *Klebsiella*, *Citrobacter*, *Proteus*, and *Serratia*. The enterococci (gram-positive aerobic non-hemolytic streptococci) may sometimes cause urosepsis. In urinary tract operations involving bowel, anaerobic bacteria may be the cause of urosepsis, and in wound infections, staphylococci, e.g., *staphylococcus aureus* and *staphylococcus epidermidis*, are the usual cause.

The recommendations for treatment of urosepsis include (Fig. 4.1; Grabe et al. 2011):

- A third-generation cephalosporin, e.g., cefotaxime intravenously (IV), ceftriaxone IV. These are active against gram-negative bacteria, but less active against staphylococci and gram-positive bacteria. Ceftazidime also has activity against *Pseudomonas aeruginosa*. It is therefore important to get an urgent gram stain on any fluid sample sent to the laboratory. About 5% of patients who are allergic to penicillin are also allergic to cephalosporins, so enquire about penicillin allergy and consider alternative antibiotics.
- Fluoroquinolones, e.g., ciprofloxacin, can be used instead of cephalosporins. They exhibit good activity against enterobacteria and *P. aeruginosa*, but less activity against staphylococci and enterococci. Ciprofloxacin can be given both orally and intravenously. It is well absorbed from the gastrointestinal tract.

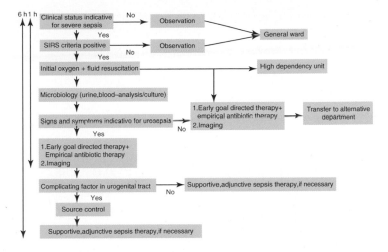

FIGURE 4.1 Clinical algorithm for the management of urosepsis (EAU guidelines; Grabe et al. (2011))

- Metronidazole is used if there is suspicion of an anaerobic source of sepsis.
- Other drugs that can be used if there is no clinical response to the above include a combination of piperacillin and tazobactam. This combination is active against enterobacteria, enterococci, and *Pseudomonas*.
- Gentamicin is used in conjunction with other antibiotics because it has a relatively narrow therapeutic spectrum (against gram-negative organisms). Close monitoring of therapeutic levels and renal function is important. It has good activity against enterobacteria and *Pseudomonas*, with poor activity against streptococci and anaerobes and therefore should ideally be combined with beta-lactam antibiotics, e.g., co-trimoxazole, but can be combined with ciprofloxacin instead.

If there is clinical improvement, intravenous treatment should continue for at least 48 h with oral medication thereafter. Make appropriate adjustments when the sensitivity results are available from the urine cultures that were sent. It may take about 48 h for sensitivity results to become available.

Pyelonephritis and Pyonephrosis

See Chap. 3.

Prostatic Infections and Prostatic Abscess

Acute Bacterial Prostatitis [National Institute of Health Classification System (Krieger et al. 1999) Category I Prostatitis]

Acute bacterial prostatitis is an infection of the prostate associated with a lower urinary tract infection and generalized sepsis. *E. coli* is the commonest cause. *Pseudomonas, Serratia, Klebsiella*, and enterococci are less common causes.

The presenting symptoms include acute onset of perineal and suprapubic pain with storage/filling (frequency, urgency, suprapubic pain) and voiding (hesitancy, poor flow, acute retention, pain on voiding) and lower urinary tract symptoms, combined with fever, chills, and malaise. The infection may be severe enough to cause septicemia.

The patient shows signs of systemic toxicity (fever, tachycardia, hypotension), combined with suprapubic tenderness and a palpable bladder, if in urinary retention. On digital rectal examination, the prostate is extremely tender.

Treatment consists of intravenous antibiotics, pain relief and relief of retention if present. Traditional teaching recommended a suprapubic catheter be inserted, rather than a urethral catheter, to avoid the potential obstruction of prostatic urethral ducts by a urethral catheter with retention of infected secretions and pus. However, in-and-out catheterization, or short periods with an indwelling catheter probably do no harm, and this is certainly an easier way of relieving retention than suprapubic catheterization.

Prostatic Abscess

Failure to respond to the treatment regimen outlined above (persistent symptoms and persistent fever while on antibiotic therapy) suggests the development of a prostatic abscess. A transrectal ultrasound, or computed tomography (CT) scan if the former proves too painful, is the best way of diagnosing a prostatic abscess (Fig. 4.2). This may be drained by a transurethral incision or de-roofing, using a resectoscope.

Fournier's Gangrene

Fournier's gangrene (Fig. 4.3) is a necrotizing fasciitis affecting the genitalia and perineum. It primarily affects males. Necrosis and subsequent gangrene of infected tissues occurs. Culture of infected tissue reveals a combination of aerobic (e.g., *E. coli*, enterococcus, *Klebsiella*) and anaerobic organisms (*Bacteroides*, *Clostridium*, microaerophilic

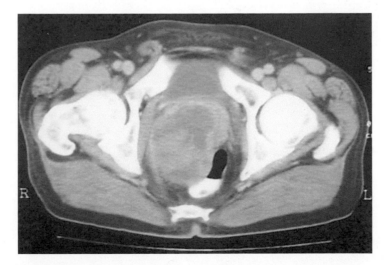

FIGURE 4.2 Prostatic abscess

streptococci), which are believed to grow in a synergistic fashion. Conditions that predispose to the development of Fournier's gangrene include diabetes, local trauma to the genitalia and perineum (e.g., zipper injuries to the foreskin), and surgical procedures such as circumcision.

Presentation

The presentation is often dramatic. A previously well patient may become systemically unwell over a very

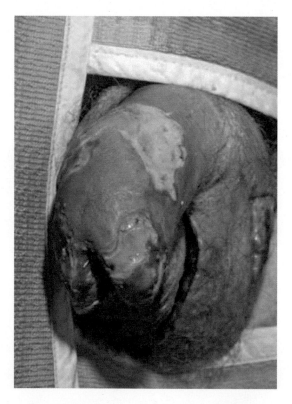

FIGURE 4.3 Fournier's gangrene

short-time course (hours) following a seemingly trivial injury to the external genitalia. A fever is usually present. The patient looks very unwell and may have marked pain in the affected tissues, and the developing sepsis may alter their mental status. The genitalia and perineum are edematous; on palpation of the affected area, there is tenderness, and crepitus may be present, indicating the presence of subcutaneous gas produced by gas-forming organisms. As the infection advances, blisters (bullae) appear in the skin and within a matter of hours, areas of necrosis may develop, which spread to involve adjacent tissues, e.g., the lower abdominal wall. The condition advances rapidly, hence its alternative name of spontaneous fulminant gangrene of the genitalia.

Although blood tests may be abnormal (e.g., elevated white count), the diagnosis is a clinical one and is based on awareness of the condition and a low index of suspicion.

Treatment

DO NOT DELAY! While intravenous access is obtained, blood is taken for culture, intravenous fluids are started and oxygen administered, and broad-spectrum antibiotics are given to cover both gram-positive and gram-negative aerobes and anaerobes, e.g., ampicillin, gentamicin, and metronidazole or clindamycin. Make arrangements to transfer the patient to the operating room as quickly as possible so that debridement of necrotic tissue (skin, subcutaneous fat) can be carried out. Extensive areas of tissue may have to be removed, but it is unusual for the testes or deeper penile tissues to be involved, and these can usually be spared. A suprapubic catheter is inserted to divert urine and allow monitoring of urine output.

Where facilities allow, consider treatment with hyperbaric oxygen therapy. There is some evidence that this may be beneficial (Pizzorno et al. 1997). Repeated debridements to remove residual necrotic tissue are not infrequently required.

Mortality is in the order of 20–30%. There is debate about whether diabetes increases the mortality rate (Chawla et al. 2003; Nisbet and Thompson 2002).

Epididymo-Orchitis

This is an inflammatory condition of the epididymis, often involving the testis, and caused by bacterial infection. It presents with pain, swelling, and tenderness of the epididymis. It should be distinguished from chronic epididymitis, where there is long-standing pain in the epididymis but usually no swelling.

Infection ascends from the urethra or bladder. In men aged <35 years, the infective organism is usually *Neisseria gonorrhea*, *Chlamydia trachomatis*, or coliform bacteria (causing a urethritis that then ascends to infect the epididymis). In children and older men, the infective organisms are usually coliforms.

A rare, non-infective cause of epididymitis is the antiarrhythmic drug amiodarone, which accumulates in high concentrations within the epididymis, causing inflammation (Gasparich et al. 1984). It can be unilateral or bilateral and resolves on discontinuation of the drug.

Differential Diagnosis

Torsion of the testicle is the main differential diagnosis. A preceding history of symptoms suggestive of urethritis or urinary infection (burning when passing urine, frequency, urgency, and suprapubic pain) suggests that epididymitis is the cause of the scrotal pain, but these symptoms may not always be present in epididymitis. In epididymitis, pain, tenderness, and swelling may be confined to the epididymis, whereas in torsion the pain and swelling are localized to the testis. However, there may be overlap in these physical signs.

Where doubt exists – where you are unsure whether you are dealing with torsion or epididymitis – exploration is the safest option. Though radionuclide scanning can differentiate between torsion and epididymitis, this is not available in many hospitals. Color Doppler ultrasonography, which provides a visual image of blood flow, can differentiate between a torsion and epididymitis, but its sensitivity for diagnosing torsion is only 80%, i.e., it misses the diagnosis of torsion in as many as 20% of cases (these 20% of cases have torsion, but normal findings on Doppler ultrasonography of the testis). Its sensitivity for diagnosing epididymitis is about 70%. Again, if in doubt, explore.

Treatment of Epididymitis

Culture the urine, any urethral discharge, and blood (if systemically unwell). Treatment consists of bed rest, analgesia, and antibiotics. Where *C. trachomatis* is a possible infecting organism, prescribe a 10- to 14-day course of tetracycline 500 mg four times a day or doxycycline 100 mg twice daily. If gonorrhea is confirmed on a gram stain of the urethral discharge (if present) and on culture, prescribe ciprofloxacin (though check the sensitivity on culture). For non-sexually transmitted disease (STD)-related epididymitis, prescribe antibiotics empirically (until culture results are available) according to your local microbiology department's advice, which will be based on local patterns of organisms isolated from urine cultures and on local patterns of antibiotic resistance. Our empirical antibiotic regimen is ciprofloxacin for 2 weeks where there is no systemic upset. When the patient is systemically unwell, we admit them for intravenous cefuroxime 1.5 gr three times a day and intravenous gentamicin 5 mg/kg, until they are apyrexial, at which time we switch to oral ciprofloxacin for 2 weeks.

Complications of Epididymitis

These include abscess formation, infarction of the testis, chronic pain, and infertility.

Periurethral Abscess

This can occur in patients with urethral stricture disease, in association with gonococcal urethritis and following urethral catheterization. These conditions predispose to bacteria (gram-negative rods, enterococci, anaerobes, gonococcus) gaining access through Buck's fascia to the periurethral tissues. If not rapidly diagnosed and treated, infection can spread to the perineum, buttocks, and abdominal wall.

The majority (90%) of patients present with scrotal swelling and a fever. Approximately 20% will have presented with urinary retention, 10% with a urethral discharge, and 10% having spontaneously discharged the abscess through the urethra. Ultrasound scanning may help in the diagnosis.

The abscess should be incised and drained, a suprapubic catheter placed to divert the urine away from the urethra, and broad-spectrum antibiotics commenced (gentamicin and cefuroxime) until antibiotic sensitivities are known.

References

Chawla SN, Gallop C, Mydlo JH. Fournier's gangrene: an analysis of repeated surgical debridement. Eur Urol. 2003;43:572–5.

Gasparich JP, Mason JT, Greene HL, et al. Non-infectious epididymitis associated with amiodarone therapy. Lancet. 1984;2:1211–2.

Grabe M, Bjerklund-Johansen TE, Botto H, et al. Guidelines on urological infections. European Association of Urology. 2011. www.uroweb.org. Accessed on March 2012.

Krieger JN, Nyberg LJ, Nickel JC. NIH consensus definition and classification of prostatitis. JAMA. 1999;282:236–7.

Nisbet AA, Thompson IM. Impact of diabetes mellitus on the presentation and outcomes of Fournier's gangrene. Urology. 2002;60:775–9.

Pizzorno R, Bonini F, Donelli A, et al. Hyperbaric oxygen therapy in the treatment of Fournier's gangrene in 100 male patients. J Urol. 1997;158:837–40.

Chapter 5
Traumatic Urological Emergencies

Noel Armenakas

Renal Injuries

Etiology

The kidney is the most frequently injured genitourinary organ, involved in up to 10 % of all civilian abdominal traumas. Overall, 65 % of genitourinary injuries involve the kidney. Most renal injuries (85–90 %) arise from *blunt* trauma. Blunt mechanisms include motor vehicle accidents, falls, and assaults and are usually low-grade injuries. The most frequently associated injuries are to the head, central nervous system, spleen, and liver. *Penetrating* injuries are usually from gunshot wounds and are almost always associated with multiple intra-abdominal organ injuries, most commonly to the liver, bowel, and spleen. Less frequent causes of penetrating renal injuries include stab wounds and percutaneous renal procedures.

N. Armenakas, M.D., FACS
Department of Urology, Lenox Hill Hospital and
New York Presbyterian Hospital (Cornell-Weill),
New York, NY, USA
e-mail: drarmenakas@nyurological.com

H. Hashim et al. (eds.), *Urological Emergencies In Clinical Practice,* DOI 10.1007/978-1-4471-2720-8_5, © Springer-Verlag London 2013

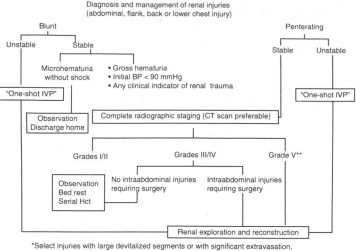

Diagnosis and management of renal injuries
(abdominal, flank, back or lower chest injury)

FIGURE 5.1 Algorithm for the diagnosis and management of renal injuries

Diagnosis (Fig. 5.1)

Renal injuries are diagnosed by combining a carefully performed *history* and *physical* examination with the appropriate *laboratory* and *radiologic* evaluation.

History

The history should provide information regarding potential renal involvement. For example, deceleration from a high-speed motor vehicle accident or a significant fall should raise a suspicion of a major vascular or parenchymal renal injury. Any penetrating trauma to the chest, abdomen, or flank is suggestive of a renal injury.

Clinical Findings

Clinical findings indicative of a potential renal injury from a blunt mechanism include:

- Flank contusions
- Seat belt marks
- Upper abdominal or flank tenderness
- Lower rib or lumbar vertebral fractures

In penetrating trauma, entry and exit wounds may suggest a transrenal course.

Initial blood pressure, recorded prior to resuscitation, is an important determinant of the likelihood of a renal injury and therefore of the need for a radiographic evaluation.

Laboratory Tests

- The urinalysis is crucial in determining the likelihood of a renal injury.
- Hematuria (defined as >5 erythrocytes per high-power field) is the hallmark of a renal injury. However, the degree of hematuria does not correlate consistently with the extent of renal injury.
- Other important laboratory tests include a complete blood count and a serum chemistry profile.

Imaging

- Radiographic imaging defines the extent of injury. It should be considered once the patient has been stabilized.
- Contrast-enhanced CT is the single best radiographic test for diagnosing renal trauma. It is noninvasive, rapid, and provides accurate detection of the renal and any associated intra-abdominal injuries.
- Intravenous pyelography was formerly the most commonly used renal imaging modality. In all major trauma centers, it

has been replaced by CT imaging because of its inferior sensitivity and the incomplete information obtained.

- Ultrasonography is limited by its inability to distinguish blood from urine, making it suboptimal for staging renal injuries. It is best used in following patients with renal injuries to avoid excess radiation exposure.
- Renal arteriography should be considered in situations where embolization is desirable in controlling bleeding.
- Magnetic resonance provides images comparable to CT. However, it is less readily available, more expensive, and more time consuming than CT, which limits its utility in a trauma setting.

Indications for Imaging

The need for radiographic renal imaging is determined by the presence of any of the following criteria (Miller and McAninch 1995):

- Any *penetrating* injury to the abdomen, flanks, back, or lower chest.
- Any *blunt* injury presenting with either of the following:
  (a) Gross hematuria
  (b) Microscopic hematuria and an initial blood pressure <90 mmHg
  (c) Any clinical indicator of renal trauma (including rapid deceleration injury or the physical findings listed above)

Patients who sustain blunt trauma and are hemodynamically stable with microscopic hematuria, in the absence of any clinical indicators of renal trauma, can be safely diagnosed with a low-grade renal injury without renal imaging.

In the hemodynamically unstable patient, where radiographic staging is not feasible, surgical staging is required. In these cases, a one-shot intravenous pyelogram (IVP) is performed 10 min after intravenous infusion of 2 ml/kg of contrast material. The primary purpose of this limited study is to assess the presence and function of the contralateral kidney.

Pediatric Renal Injuries

Pediatric renal injuries are evaluated similarly, except that a further distinction is made regarding the degree of microhematuria with blunt trauma only. Specifically, a finding of >50 erythrocytes per high-power field warrants radiographic imaging (Morey et al. 1996).

Injury Classification (Fig. 5.2)

On the basis of the radiographic and/or clinical information obtained, renal injuries are classified according to severity into five grades:

Grade I: contusion or subcapsular hematoma
Grade II: <1 cm parenchymal laceration
Grade III: >1 cm parenchymal laceration without urinary extravasation
Grade IV: deep parenchymal laceration with urinary extravasation or a contained vascular injury
Grade V: shattered kidney or avulsion of the renal pedicle

Management
(Matthews et al. 1997; Toutouzas et al. 2002)
(Fig. 5.1)

Most renal injuries are now managed conservatively. This changing paradigm has evolved as a consequence of improved injury staging with CT, successful experience managing other solid abdominal organ injuries (e.g., splenic and liver lacerations), and the judicious use of ancillary procedures (e.g., angiography, percutaneous drainage, ureteral stenting).

- Nonoperative management has become the standard of care for most grade I–IV renal injuries from a blunt mechanism; grade V injuries are best managed surgically.

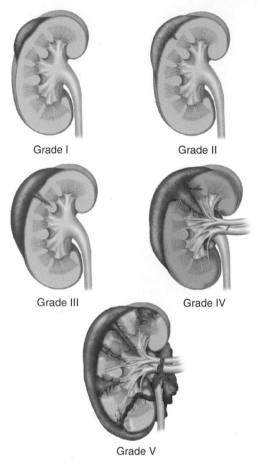

Grade I

Grade II

Grade III

Grade IV

Grade V

FIGURE 5.2 Grading system for renal injuries. American Association for the Surgery of Trauma Organ Injury Severity Scale

- Most low-grade penetrating renal injuries (grades I, II) can be observed. High-grade penetrating renal injuries (grades III–V) usually have associated intra-abdominal organ injuries requiring laparotomy and should be explored and reconstructed.
- Overall, approximately 95 % of blunt and more than 50 % of penetrating renal injuries can be safely managed nonoperatively.

- Percutaneous angiographic techniques are becoming increasingly important in managing renal injuries. Selective arterial embolization can be used to control both acute and delayed renal bleeding, as an adjunct to nonoperative management. They can be particularly useful in managing iatrogenic renal hemorrhage from a renal biopsy or Percutaneous nephrolithotomy (PCNL), as well as delayed bleeding from any major blunt or penetrating injury. CT findings that may predict the need for angiographic embolization include the size of the perirenal hematoma (>3.5 cm) and the presence of intravascular extravasation of contrast material (Nuss et al. 2009).

Renal Exploration

Although most renal injuries do not require intervention, when surgery is indicated, it should be performed expeditiously and carefully. Indications for renal exploration are listed in Table 5.1. The goal of renal exploration is to control bleeding. Every attempt should be made to preserve the kidney, providing it is safe to do so. In cases of renal pedicle avulsion, a nephrectomy should be performed as a lifesaving measure.

The following principles apply for renal exploration:

- A traumatized kidney should be explored through a midline transperitoneal incision extending from the xiphoid process to the pubic symphysis.

TABLE 5.1 Indications for renal exploration

Absolute:
Hemodynamic instability from renal hemorrhage suggested by an expanding or pulsatile retroperitoneal hematoma
Relative:
Urinary extravasation
>25 % nonviable renal parenchyma
Renovascular injury
Persistent bleeding (>2 units transfused per 24 h)
Incomplete radiographic staging
Laparotomy for associated injuries

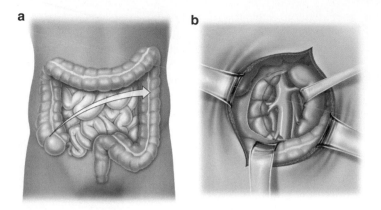

FIGURE 5.3 (**a**) Transverse colon and small bowel retracted. (**b**) Posterior peritoneal window exposing the renal vessels

- An exploratory laparotomy should be performed to inspect the entire intra-abdominal contents.
- Early renal vascular control is advised to allow for immediate vascular occlusion in cases of massive hemorrhage. This is achieved by retracting the transverse colon and small bowel superiorly and placing them on the patient's chest (Fig. 5.3a). A retroperitoneal incision is made over the abdominal aorta and extended cephalad to the ligament of Treitz. A posterior peritoneal window is created, exposing the renal vessels which are isolated and secured with vessel loops (Fig. 5.3b). In cases where an extensive retroperitoneal hematoma obscures palpation of the abdominal aorta, the retroperitoneal incision is made medial to the inferior mesenteric vein.

Renal Reconstruction

General principles of renal reconstruction include:

- Broad exposure of the entire kidney
- Debridement of nonviable parenchyma
- Meticulous hemostasis
- Adequate closure of the collecting system

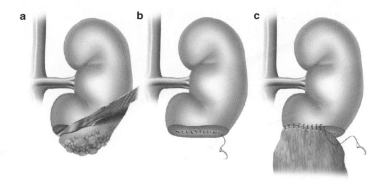

FIGURE 5.4 Partial nephrectomy following renal trauma. (**a**) Partial (polar) nephrectomy. (**b**) Closure of the collecting system. (**c**) Omental advancement flap

- Reapproximation of the parenchymal edges (renorrhaphy)
- Perirenal drainage, where appropriate

Parenchymal Injuries

Upper and lower pole renal injuries can be managed with partial nephrectomy, whereas a renorrhaphy suffices for most mid-renal injuries (Figs. 5.4 and 5.5). In either case, the collecting system should be closed and bleeding parenchymal vessels ligated with 3–0 or 4–0 absorbable sutures (chromic gut). The renal defect should be loosely approximated with 2–0 monofilament absorbable sutures (polydioxanone or polyglyconate) and appropriately covered. An absorbable gelatin sponge bolster (Gelfoam) alone or in conjunction with an omental flap can be used to cover the defect. Additionally, hemostatic matrix (e.g., Floseal or Surgiflo) may be helpful in securing the closure and minimizing bleeding.

Vascular Injuries

A major injury to the main renal vessels usually requires prompt operative management. Vascular occlusion is necessary when attempting repair. Repair of major injuries to the main

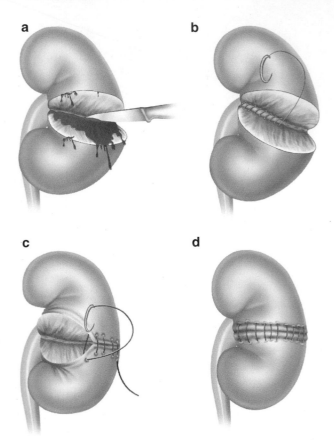

FIGURE 5.5 Renorrhaphy technique. (**a**) Deep mid-renal laceration. (**b**) Closure of the renal pelvis and ligation of any bleeding parenchymal vessels. (**c**) Renal defect closure. (**d**) Completed renorrhaphy over a gelatin sponge bolster

renal artery should be reserved for solitary or bilaterally injured kidneys. Successful renal salvage after major renovascular injury occurs in less than 35 % of cases (Tillou et al. 2001).

Partial renovascular lacerations can be repaired with running 5–0 vascular sutures (Fig. 5.6). The left renal vein can be safely ligated because of collateral drainage pro-

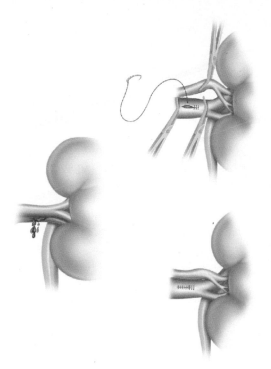

FIGURE 5.6 Technique of suturing a laceration of the main renal vein

vided by the adrenal and gonadal veins. Similarly, injured segmental renal vessels can be ligated; with arterial ligation, this will result in devascularized renal tissue, which is usually inconsequential.

Drainage

Drains should be used liberally in cases of collecting system or associated intra-abdominal organ involvement. Either a passive (Penrose) or a suction (Jackson-Pratt) drain is appropriate. Typically, the drain is maintained for 72 h or until the output decreases sufficiently.

Complications

Early

- *Persistent bleeding* which should initially be managed with bed rest and the appropriate resuscitative techniques (i.e., hydration, close monitoring of vital signs and hematocrit, and transfusion, if needed). In hemodynamically unstable patients or when multiple transfusions are required, angiography should be considered. In such cases, selective arteriographic embolization usually controls the bleeding, but more than one procedure may be needed to achieve hemostasis. When delayed exploration is required to control hemorrhage, the nephrectomy rate is >50 %.
- *Urinary extravasation* leading to a urinoma, infection, or abscess. This is caused by a persistent collecting system leak. The diagnosis is made by abdominal CT or renal sonography. The mainstay of treatment is adequate percutaneous drainage and appropriate antibiotic coverage. A ureteral double-J stent may be helpful for persistent extravasation. Urinary leaks almost always resolve spontaneously.

Delayed

- *Delayed bleeding* usually occurs within the first 3 weeks of injury. Management is similar to early persistent bleeding.
- *Arteriovenous (AV) fistulae* usually occur after percutaneous renal procedures. Their incidence after renal biopsy may be as high as 15 %. Most are inconsequential and resolve spontaneously. Symptomatic AV fistulas (causing persistent bleeding or hypertension) can be treated with arteriographic localization and selective embolization.
- *Hypertension* is caused by either renovascular injury (leading to arteriovenous fistula, arterial thrombosis, or stenosis) or renal parenchymal compression (from extravasated blood or urine producing a Page kidney). The physiologic mechanism is through stimulation of the renin-angiotensin system

by partial renal ischemia. This usually occurs within the first year of injury. The true incidence of posttraumatic hypertension is unknown with reported ranges from 0 to 30 %.

- *Decreased renal function* is related to the degree of injury and its sequelae. Extensive areas of devitalized renal parenchyma and renovascular injuries have a higher likelihood of significant reduction in renal function.

Complications of angiographic embolization include the following: clot dislodgment (causing additional bleeding), arterial dissection, coil migration, segmental renal necrosis, and contrast-induced renal insufficiency.

Outcome

Aggressive, accurate staging of renal trauma is important in avoiding renal loss. Although most renal injuries can be managed nonoperatively, renal salvage can be achieved in the majority of cases requiring exploration, providing the correct steps are followed and with the proper expertise.

Bleeding Post-Renal Surgery

Etiology

The etiology of a bleed, in a postsurgical setting, is usually clear as it is a consequence of the procedure performed. The most common cause of an iatrogenic perirenal bleed is a percutaneous renal biopsy. Radiographic evidence of bleeding is identified in up to 60 % of these cases (Ginsburg et al. 1980). Most are inconsequential, do not require any intervention, and heal spontaneously. Other renal surgical procedures that can result in postoperative hemorrhage are listed in Table 5.2. Mechanisms of injury include a dislodged vascular clip or suture, direct vascular or parenchymal laceration, intimal dissection, arteriovenous fistula, and pseudoaneurysm. The origin of the bleed can be venous, arterial, or both. Besides the kidney itself, other

TABLE 5.2   Renal surgical procedures causing bleeding

Open or laparoscopic renal surgery

  Partial nephrectomy

  Total nephrectomy

  Cyst decortication

Percutaneous renal surgery

  Nephrolithotomy

  Resection of upper tract urothelial tumors

  Endopyelotomy

  Cryosurgery

  Radiofrequency ablation

Renovascular surgery

  Angioplasty and stent placement

Renal biopsy

sources of bleeding include the spleen, liver, or adjacent vessels.

This is in contrast to a spontaneous renal hemorrhage, which is often multifactorial. Precipitating factors include an undiagnosed renal tumor (malignant or angiomyolipoma), anticoagulation, and underlying hematologic disorders (such as leukemia, hemophilia, thrombocytopenia, and antiphospholipid antibody syndrome). Any of these complicating factors can obscure the evaluation and treatment of postoperative renal bleeding.

Diagnosis

Open or Laparoscopic Surgery

The diagnosis of a renal bleed should be considered in any patient after open or laparoscopic renal surgery. In most cases, the presentation is acute. Delayed bleeding can occur within the first 2–3 weeks of surgery.

- Symptoms include a sudden increase in abdominal or flank pain which may be associated with nausea and vomiting.
- Clinical signs include hypovolemia, tachycardia, hypotension, and pallor.
- Hematuria and increased sanguineous drainage from the incision or drain site are common findings.
- On physical examination, the abdomen may be distended and tender with voluntary guarding and hypoactive bowel sounds.
- Serum laboratory findings include a falling hemoglobin and hematocrit, and leukocytosis.

Contrast-enhanced CT is the initial imaging modality used to identify the degree and source of bleeding. Dynamic sequential images, taken within 1 min of intravenous contrast administration, provide optimal vascular detail. Conventional CT images can then be used to assess renal parenchymal and perirenal anatomy as well as renal excretion.

Percutaneous Renal Surgery

Bleeding during percutaneous renal surgery can occur during any part of the procedure, including renal access, dilation, nephroscopy, or intrarenal surgery. Most commonly, bleeding is caused by inadvertent injury to the segmental arteries. A transparenchymal posterolateral approach provides the safest access to the collecting system for percutaneous surgery. During endopyelotomy, bleeding may be caused by injury to an anomalous crossing vessel or variant vasculature.

The diagnosis of renal bleeding during percutaneous renal surgery is usually made clinically by seeing a sudden gush of blood from the puncture or nephrostomy site. Delayed hemorrhage occurs in approximately 1 % of patients and is usually due to an arteriovenous fistula or arterial pseudoaneurysm (Kessaris et al. 1995). For persistent uncontrollable bleeding, angiography rather than CT is used because of its dual diagnostic and therapeutic role. Angiographic findings include arteriovenous fistula, arterial pseudoaneurysm, and contrast extravasation suggesting a vascular laceration. Occasionally, multiple vascular injuries can be encountered.

Management

Initial Management

Primary management involves stabilization of the patient and assessment of the degree and rapidity of bleeding using the appropriate clinical, laboratory, and radiographic means. Initial resuscitative measures include restoration of intravascular volume with intravenous fluids and transfusion of blood products, including fresh frozen plasma, clotting factors, and platelets, where necessary. Any underlying hematologic disorder should be identified and corrected. Venous hemorrhage usually responds to such conservative management.

Bleeding encountered during percutaneous renal surgery should be managed initially with placement of a larger sheath or an appropriate nephrostomy catheter in order to compress the renal parenchyma. In addition, the catheter can be clamped to facilitate clotting of the collecting system. If bleeding persists, despite these simple occlusive maneuvers, additional intervention may be required.

Intervention
(Kessaris et al. 1995; Baumann et al. 2007; Richstone et al. 2008)

The need for intervention is determined by the initial evaluation and the patient's response to conservative management.

Angioembolization

In cases of intractable bleeding, angiography with embolization is the procedure of choice. The goal of embolization is to selectively completely occlude any bleeding vessel(s) while limiting collateral parenchymal damage which can lead to segmental renal necrosis. This is accomplished by identifying the cause of hemorrhage (including bleeding vessels, arteriovenous fistulas, pseudoaneurysms) and performing superselective embolization. Angioembolization usually suffices in controlling bleeding, although more than one procedure may be required.

Laparotomy

In cases where angioembolization has failed to control bleeding resulting in hemodynamic deterioration, surgical exploration should be performed via a laparotomy. The first step is to evacuate the hematoma and identify the source of bleeding. Direct manual compression of the bleeding site and appropriate use of packing will facilitate visualization. Renal bleeding can usually be controlled effectively with fine absorbable sutures and reinforced with a hemostatic matrix (e.g., Floseal or Surgiflo). Placement of clips or sutures blindly is discouraged as it can worsen the situation. A vascular surgery consult may be necessary to assist in cases involving the major vessels. For splenic injuries, an emergent splenectomy may be required. Most hepatic injuries can be managed with precise suturing and use of the appropriate hemostatic matrix. In cases of persistent renal bleeding in a compromised patient, an expedient nephrectomy is often the safest option.

Complications

The most common complication of post-renal surgery hemorrhage is the loss of renal function. Other complications include pseudoaneurysm, arteriovenous fistula, infection, and hypertension.

Outcome

Postoperative renal hemorrhage should be suspected in any patient after recent renal surgery. If initial conservative management fails to control the bleeding, superselective angiographic embolization should be performed expeditiously and cautiously in an effort to preserve renal function. In rare cases, where embolization is unsuccessful in controlling bleeding, an emergent exploratory laparotomy should be performed. In such situations, a nephrectomy may be an essential lifesaving maneuver.

Acute Renal Artery Occlusion

Acute renal artery occlusion can occur from thrombi or emboli. The major concern is the development of irreversible renal damage. In experimental models, renal viability is lost after complete vascular occlusion of >3 h. Renal arterial thrombosis commonly involves the proximal or middle third of the main renal artery, whereas renal artery embolization usually involves the peripheral arterial branches. Both are more common on the left side because of the shorter and more acutely angulated left renal artery.

Etiology

- Renal artery thrombi result from platelet adhesion and aggregation following damage to the arterial endothelium.
- Renal artery emboli usually originate in the heart and travel downstream where they lodge in the renal vessels.
- Iatrogenic causes of renal artery occlusion have increased following endovascular aortic and renovascular procedures. The risk of a major complication associated with renal artery procedures is 7–10 % (Isles et al. 1999).

The causes of renal artery occlusion are listed in Table 5.3.

Diagnosis

History

Acute renal artery occlusion should be suspected in any patient with a history of increased risk for renovascular disease presenting with the any clinical or laboratory findings suggesting ischemia. In addition, blunt abdominal trauma from a rapid deceleration, such as a high-speed motor vehicle accident or a fall, may be associated with renal artery occlusion.

TABLE 5.3 Etiology of renal artery embolism and thrombosis

Spontaneous

Cardiovascular

   Atrial fibrillation

   Bacterial endocarditis

   Renal artery aneurysm

   Acute myocardial infarction

   Hypertension

   Atherosclerosis

Autoimmune

   Polyarteritis nodosum

   Systemic lupus

   Fibromuscular dysplasia

Acquired

Trauma

Angiography/angioplasty

Open heart surgery

Neonatal umbilical artery catheterization

Clinical Findings

- There are no signs or symptoms specific to renal artery occlusion.
- Patients with *chronic* unilateral renal artery occlusion are usually asymptomatic.
- With *acute* unilateral renal artery occlusion, the most common presenting findings are abdominal and costovertebral angle tenderness and can be of varying intensities. Additional findings include nausea, fever, and hypertension.

- Severe oliguria or anuria suggests bilateral renal artery occlusion.
- Often, the diagnosis is missed early because of the more common differential diagnoses considered, including gastroenteritis, renal colic, pyelonephritis, cholecystitis, pancreatitis, and myocardial infarction.

Laboratory Tests

Serum

- Elevated lactate dehydrogenase (LDH)
- Elevated creatinine kinase (CK)
- Leukocytosis

Urine

- Microhematuria
- Proteinuria

Radiographic Tests

- CT with intravenous contrast provides the most reliable and expedient information in patients suspected of having a renal artery occlusion.
- Alternate imaging tests include magnetic resonance angiography (MRA) and angiography (which are more time consuming) and nuclear renal scans and ultrasonography with color Doppler (which are less sensitive and more difficult to interpret).
- Characteristic radiographic findings include a lack of renal parenchymal enhancement and absence of contrast excretion.
- Additional radiographic findings include renal hematomas, contrast extravasation, or a filling defect in the renal artery.
- A "cortical rim sign" may be noted which is attributed to capsular cortical perfusion (Fig. 5.7).

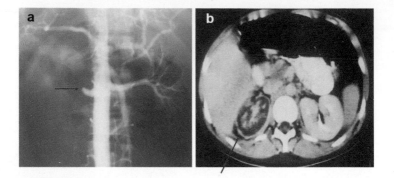

FIGURE 5.7 (**a**) Arteriography showing right renal artery occlusion from a thrombus after blunt abdominal trauma (*arrow*). (**b**) The same patients' CT scan with a right renal cortical "rim sign" from capsular vessels (*arrow*) (Images courtesy of Allen Morey, M.D.)

Management

Prompt diagnosis and treatment are critical in limiting irreversible renal damage in patients with acute renal artery occlusion. Nonoperative management is advised in patients with unilateral occlusion with surgery limited selectively to patients with a solitary kidney or bilateral renal involvement. Stabilization of renal function is best achieved in patients with partial renal artery occlusion treated within 3 h of the insult (Blum et al. 1993). Complete occlusions or partial occlusions with a delay in diagnosis fair poorly with any of the available treatments.

The appropriate elective thorough medical evaluation of all patients with spontaneous renal artery occlusion should be performed to identify an underlying cause and intervene accordingly.

Nonoperative Management

- Spontaneous renal arterial occlusion suggests underlying extra renal disease and is best managed nonoperatively with systemic anticoagulation or percutaneous thromboembolectomy.

- Medical management includes anticoagulants and thrombolytics (streptokinase, urokinase, or tissue-type plasminogen activator), administered systemically or by percutaneous transcatheterization.

Operative Management

- Operative techniques include open thromboembolectomy, bypass grafting, and autotransplantation.
- Most successful revascularizations are performed within 6 h of the occlusion (Spirnak and Resnick 1987).

Complications

The primary complication of renal artery occlusion is renal ischemia with irreversible loss of renal function. This can result in renal insufficiency and renovascular hypertension. Additional short-term complications include renal hemorrhage and infection.

Outcome

Renal artery occlusions are difficult to diagnose and require prompt intervention to preserve renal function. These limitations result in poor outcomes overall. Duration and degree of renal artery occlusion are important factors in predicting outcome. The shorter the duration of ischemia and the lesser the degree of occlusion, the greater the chance of renal preservation.

Renal Vein Thrombosis

Renal vein thrombosis occurs in two subpopulations: neonates and adults. In neonates, it usually presents within a few days of birth. In adults, it is usually associated with nephrotic syndrome. The thrombus often begins in the small venous tributaries of the renal parenchyma and propagates to the main renal vein. It may be unilateral or bilateral and can extend to the vena cava.

Etiology

The causes of renal vein thrombosis are listed in Table 5.4.

TABLE 5.4 Etiology of renal vein thrombosis

Neonatal renal vein thrombosis

    Severe dehydration (from diarrhea or vomiting)

    Maternal diabetes mellitus

    Perinatal distress

    Traumatic delivery

    Hypotension

    Cardiac disease

Adult renal vein thrombosis

    Nephrotic syndrome

    Trauma

    Oral contraceptives

    Steroid administration

    Renal transplantation

    Renal tumors

Neonatal Renal Vein Thrombosis

The pathophysiology is thought to be a decrease in renal blood flow occurring in the newborn with maternal or fetal risk factors for thrombus formation.

Adult Renal Vein Thrombosis

- Renal vein thrombosis often occurs in the setting of the nephrotic syndrome. It is the consequence of a hypercoagulable state created by the alteration of various coagulation components.
- Membranous nephropathy is the most common underlying nephropathy associated with renal vein thrombosis, occurring in approximately two-thirds of cases (Laville et al. 1988). Other less common, predisposing nephropathies include membranoproliferative glomerulonephritis, lipoid nephrosis, amyloidosis, renal sarcoidosis, and lupus nephritis (Llach et al. 1977).

Diagnosis

History

The diagnosis should be suspected in any patient with a history suggestive of an increased risk of renal vein thrombosis. It is often missed, especially in cases of unilateral thrombosis and a normally functioning contralateral kidney.

Clinical Findings

Neonatal Renal Vein Thrombosis

The most common clinical finding is an enlarged palpable kidney (in 60 %). Other findings include oliguria, anuria, and cardiovascular shock.

Adult Renal Vein Thrombosis

Often patients are asymptomatic. This is particularly true with chronic thrombosis. Patients presenting acutely may complain of sudden flank pain and on exam will have marked costovertebral angle tenderness. Peripheral edema occurs with the nephrotic syndrome.

Laboratory Tests

Neonatal Renal Vein Thrombosis

- Common laboratory findings include hematuria, thrombocytopenia, and acidosis.

Adult Renal Vein Thrombosis

- Serum: hypoalbuminemia, elevated fibrinogen and protein C, thrombocytosis
- Urine: hematuria, proteinuria

Radiographic Tests

Neonatal Renal Vein Thrombosis

- Whenever possible, color Doppler ultrasonography should be used exclusively to confirm the diagnosis, avoiding excessive radiation from CT or venacavography in neonates.

Adult Renal Vein Thrombosis

- CT with intravenous contrast is the preferred imaging test for the evaluation of renal vein thrombosis in adults. Characteristic findings include an increase in the renal vein diameter or a low-attenuation venous filling defect.
- Initially, the kidney appears enlarged with prolongation of the vascular phase. Over time, the kidney will decrease in size and progress to atrophy.

- An additional radiographic finding may be ureteral notching occurring from compression by dilated collateral veins.
- Extension of the thrombus into the vena cava is not uncommon. Pulmonary emboli may also be associated with renal vein thrombosis.
- In select cases, inferior vena cavography with selective catheterization and/or renal arteriography may be needed to confirm the diagnosis.
- Color Doppler ultrasonography can be helpful in assessing venous flow velocity, but may be less reliable than the other invasive imaging modalities.

Management

Neonatal Renal Vein Thrombosis

- Prompt resuscitation constitutes the initial management. This includes restoration of fluid and electrolyte imbalances, correction of acidosis, and assessment of cardiovascular and renal status.
- Anticoagulant therapy is required for bilateral thrombosis; its role in unilateral disease is less clear.

Adult Renal Vein Thrombosis

- The mainstay of management is anticoagulant therapy. Initially, heparin is administered at a dose needed to maintain clotting times of 2–2.5 normal. Oral anticoagulants are started after several days and continued long term. In the acute setting, anticoagulant therapy can achieve recanalization of the renal vein or even complete clot dissolution. In chronic situations, the objective is to reduce the occurrence of new thromboembolic episodes.
- Dialysis may be required for bilateral disease.
- Thrombolytic therapy and surgical thrombectomy are rarely indicated.
- Percutaneous mechanical thrombectomy can be used in select cases.

Complications

The most common complications of renal vein thrombosis include renal failure, hemorrhage, infection, and hypertension.

Outcome

The rapidity of the venous occlusion and the development of venous collateral circulation determine the clinical presentation and subsequent outcome. In general, anticoagulation appears to improve long-term renal outcome. The prognosis for patients with nephrotic syndrome with renal vein thrombosis is poor and is determined by the presence or absence of recurrent thrombotic complications. Follow-up of neonates suggests an increase in renal atrophy and hypertension (Zigman et al. 2000).

Ureteral Injuries

Etiology

External Trauma
(Perez-Brayfield et al. 2001; Elliot and McAninch 2003)

Ureteral injuries comprise up to 3 % of all genitourinary injuries from external trauma. Most are *penetrating* injuries from gunshot wounds and are almost always associated with multiple organ injuries, most commonly to the small intestine, colon, liver, and iliac vessels. Ureteral injuries from *blunt* trauma are rare. The mechanism is usually a rapid deceleration, occurring in children or adolescents, which results in disruption of the ureteropelvic junction. Such injuries are most commonly associated with injuries to the liver, spleen, and skeletal system.

Iatrogenic Trauma
(Assimos et al. 1994; Frankman et al. 2010)

Overall, the most common cause of ureteral trauma is iatrogenic. Intraoperative mechanisms of ureteral injury include transection, avulsion, resection, crush, devascularization, electrocoagulation, and suture ligation.

- Ureteroscopic procedures are the most frequent causes of iatrogenic ureteral trauma. Most are minor (such as mucosal false passages or perforations) and are usually inconsequential. Major injuries include avulsions and intussusceptions. The incidence of ureteroscopic ureteral injuries has decreased with the use of smaller-caliber endoscopes.
- Most significant ureteral injuries occur during gynecologic procedures, including:
  - Hysterectomy (total abdominal, radical, vaginal)
  - Cesarean section
  - Oophorectomy

- Other operations during which the ureter may be injured include:

  - General surgical procedures (low anterior resection and abdominal perineal resection)
  - Vascular procedures (aortoiliac and aortofemoral arterial bypass surgery)
  - Spinal and orthopedic surgeries

Factors that predispose to iatrogenic ureteral trauma are listed in Table 5.5.

Awareness of the ureter's anatomical course and the areas of greatest susceptibility to trauma is important in preventing iatrogenic injuries. The use of intraoperative stents in indentifying the ureters and preventing inadvertent injury has been evaluated extensively. Although intuitively ureteral stenting prior to a major abdominopelvic operation can aid in tactile ureteral localization and possibly injury avoidance and recognition, a clear advantage has not been established (Chou et al. 2009). In general, universal routine stenting prior to major abdominopelvic procedures is not advised.

TABLE 5.5 Factors that predispose to iatrogenic ureteral injury

Prior surgery
Infection of inflammation (diverticulitis, pelvic inflammatory disease, endometriosis)
Radiation therapy
Malignancy
Uterine size >12 weeks gestation
Ovarian mass >4 cm
Obesity
Massive bleeding
Congenital anomalies (ureteral duplication, retrocaval ureter, horseshoe kidney)

Diagnosis (Fig. 5.8)

Prompt diagnosis is the first step toward a successful outcome. With external ureteral trauma, this is complicated by the presence of multiple organ injuries and the absence of early clinical and laboratory findings specific for ureteral trauma. Iatrogenic injuries caused by devascularization or coagulation are particularly prone to a delay in diagnosis as the injury can evolve slowly. In general, all ureteral injuries can be difficult to diagnose and require a high index of suspicion.

Clinical Findings

- Early clinical indicators of ureteral trauma are vague or nonexistent.
- Delayed signs or symptoms of a ureteral injury include prolonged ileus, persistent flank pain, fever, urinary obstruction, urinary leakage, fistula formation, anuria, and eventually sepsis.

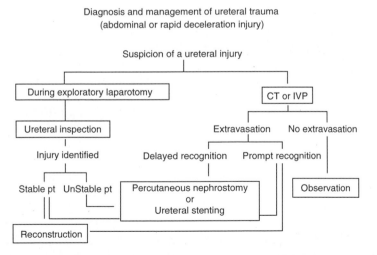

FIGURE 5.8 Algorithm for the diagnosis and management of ureteral injuries

- Overall, more than 90 % of ureteral injuries from external trauma are identified immediately, whereas less than half of iatrogenic ureteral injuries are recognized promptly.
- Any patient with penetrating or blunt abdominal trauma to the flank or abdomen or after abdominal or pelvic surgery, presenting with signs or symptoms suggestive of a possible ureteral injury, should be thoroughly evaluated either radiographically or intraoperatively.

Laboratory Findings

- Hematuria is absent in approximately 30 % of ureteral injuries from an external mechanism.
- With delayed diagnosis, azotemia may be the only finding.

Imaging

- Contrast-enhanced CT is the preferred imaging test for ureteral injuries. Delayed films should be obtained to ensure adequate visualization during the excretory CT phase. Medial extravasation of contrast with absence of distal ureteral opacification on delayed images is diagnostic of a complete ureteral disruption.
- Retrograde ureteropyelography provides the best images of the ureter, but is not always practical in an acutely polytraumatized patient as it adds time to an already precarious situation and requires additional equipment (e.g., fluoroscopy, cystoscopy). In an elective setting, a retrograde ureteropyelogram should be performed. This is advised when evaluating any iatrogenic ureteral injury.
- Intravenous pyelography can be used if no other imaging modality is available. It has an accuracy of approximately 70 %. A negative study should not prevent surgical exploration of the ureter when an injury is suspected.
- Contrast extravasation is the radiographic *sine qua non* of a ureteral injury.

Intraoperative Evaluation

- During a laparotomy or laparoscopy, ureteral integrity can be assessed visually and aided by injection of methylene blue or indigo carmine dyes intravenously or intraureterally (via an angiocatheter).
- Urinary leakage and extravasation of dye are clear signs of a ureteral injury.
- Ureteral discoloration and decreased ureteral peristalsis are more subtle findings which may suggest a ureteral injury.
- During cystoscopy, the ureteral efflux of dye from both ureters excludes a complete ureteral transection, but not a partial ureteral transection or contusion.
- Ureteral catheters can be passed either cystoscopically or through a cystotomy. A ureteral injury is unlikely with easy catheter passage. It is important to evaluate both ureters.

Injury Classification

Ureteral injuries are classified on the basis of radiographic or intraoperative findings, as follows:

Grade I: contusion or hematoma without devascularization

Grade II: <50 % transection

Grade III: >50 % transection

Grade IV: complete transection with >2 cm devascularization

Grade V: avulsion with >2 cm devascularization

Management (Fig. 5.8)

Selection of the appropriate management depends on the patient's condition, promptness in injury recognition, and the grade of injury.

External Trauma

- Most patients with ureteral injuries from an external mechanism require prompt operative exploration for management of their associated abdominal injuries which take precedence over the ureteral injury.
- If identified intraoperatively, in a stable patient, the injured ureter should be promptly repaired.
- Ureteral injuries with a significant delay in diagnosis or in an unstable patient are best managed initially by urinary diversion (via a percutaneous nephrostomy or ureteral stent) or creation of a cutaneous ureterostomy. Subsequent reconstruction can be scheduled electively.
- During surgery on a severely injured patient, the lethal triad of acidosis, hypothermia, and coagulopathy require a *damage control* approach. This involves termination of the surgical procedure with transfer to the intensive care unit for aggressive hemodynamic and physiologic resuscitation. The patient is then returned to the operating room, after 24–36 h, for definitive repair of their injuries (including ureteral reconstruction).

Iatrogenic Trauma

- There is a delay in diagnosing most non-urological iatrogenic injuries.
- Initial management usually involves urinary diversion alone.
- After completion of the retrograde ureteropyelogram, a gentle attempt can be made at retrograde ureteral stenting. If a stent cannot be easily passed, the urine should be diverted through a percutaneous nephrostomy.
- *Many of these injuries will heal with urinary diversion alone* (Lask et al. 1995; Ku et al. 2003).

Ureteral Reconstruction

Ureteral exploration is best performed through a midline abdominal incision. In delayed ureteral reconstruction, the incision can be tailored to the specific procedure, for example,

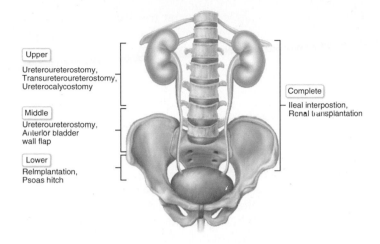

FIGURE 5.9 Options for ureteral reconstruction by level of injury

a subcostal incision can be used for upper and mid-ureteral injuries and a Gibson (muscle-splitting) incision for lower ureteral injuries. Most ureteral injuries are reconstructed using open surgical techniques. With advances in laparoscopic and robotic surgery, experience is emerging using these minimally invasive techniques to reconstruct the ureter. With concomitant intra-abdominal organ injuries, a greater omental flap can be used to exclude the ureter and protect the repair.

General principles of ureteral reconstruction include:

- Careful debridement
- Creation of a watertight tension-free repair (using absorbable sutures)
- Isolation from surrounding organs
- Adequate ureteral and retroperitoneal drainage

Specific reconstructive techniques are dependent on the location and extent of injury and are summarized in Fig. 5.9.

Ureteral Suture Ligation and Partial Ureteral Transection

Select minor iatrogenic ureteral injuries that are identified intraoperatively and felt to be due either to inadvertent ureteral ligation or a clean partial transection can be managed simply by suture removal or primary closure, respectively. The ureter must be observed carefully for any signs of devascularization, and a ureteral stent is placed.

Distal Ureteral Injuries

Ureteroneocystostomy (Fig. 5.10)

Injuries to the distal third of the ureter are best managed by submucosal bladder reimplantation. This is usually done with a combined intravesical and extravesical approach, bringing the ureter through the posterior bladder wall just medial to the original hiatus. Where possible, a submucosal tunnel can be created based on the standard 3:1 ratio (tunnel length to ureteral diameter). Ensuring a tension-free anastomosis supersedes creation of a tunneled reconstruction, as reflux in an adult patient is usually inconsequential.

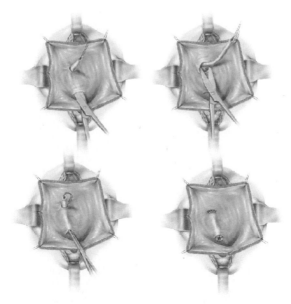

FIGURE 5.10 Ureteral reimplantation using an intra- and extravesical approach

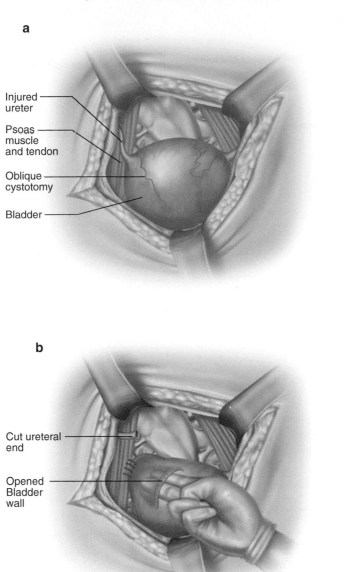

FIGURE 5.11 Psoas hitch reconstruction. (**a**) Distal ureteral identification. (**b**) Bladder mobilization. (**c**) Ureteral reimplantation and bladder closure

c

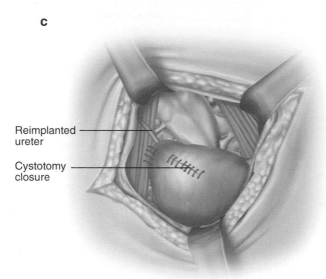

Reimplanted
ureter

Cystotomy
closure

FIGURE 5. 11 (continued)

Psoas Hitch (Fig. 5.11)

Injuries to the entire lower third of the ureter are best
managed with a psoas hitch in conjunction with ureteral
reimplantation. The bladder fundus is mobilized by dissecting it away from the peritoneal reflection. The contralateral
superior vesical pedicle is ligated. When necessary, bilateral
superior pedicle ligation affords improved bladder mobilization. An oblique anterior cystotomy is made perpendicular to
the involved ureter. The bladder dome is then guided over
the ipsilateral iliac vessels and anchored to the psoas tendon,
with interrupted sutures, taking care not to entrap the gen-
itofemoral nerve. The ureter is reimplanted, as previously
described, and the bladder wall closed perpendicular to the
cystotomy in two layers, leaving a suprapubic tube for
drainage.

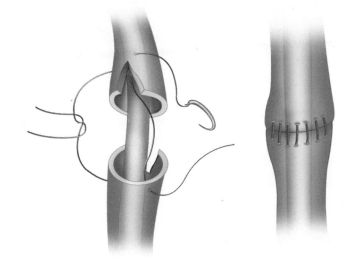

FIGURE 5.12 Primary ureteroureterostomy

Middle and Upper Ureteral Injuries

Ureteroureterostomy (Fig. 5.12)

Most grade II to IV transections involving the middle or upper third of the ureter are best managed by a primary ureteroureterostomy. The ureteral ends are carefully dissected and debrided. Each end is spatulated on opposite sides, and a watertight tension-free anastomosis is fashioned over a ureteral stent using fine absorbable sutures (4–0 chromic).

Boari Flap (Fig. 5.13)

Injuries encompassing the lower two-thirds of the ureter are best managed with an anterior bladder wall flap, in conjunction with a psoas hitch. This procedure should be used cautiously in patients with prior pelvic irradiation and avoided in the presence of neurogenic bladder disease with limited bladder capacity. The bladder is mobilized (as previously described),

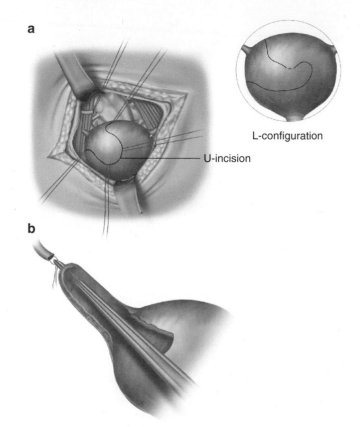

FIGURE 5.13 Boari flap. (**a**) Creation of a U- or L-shaped anterior bladder wall flap. (**b**) Submucosal ureteral reimplantation

and a full-thickness, U-shaped incision is made in its anterior wall; for longer defects, additional length can be obtained using an L-shaped configuration. The flap is raised toward the involved ureter, and the bladder wall hitched to the psoas tendon. The ureter is reimplanted submucosally into the flap, which is then closed in a tubularized configuration. Bladder closure is completed in two layers.

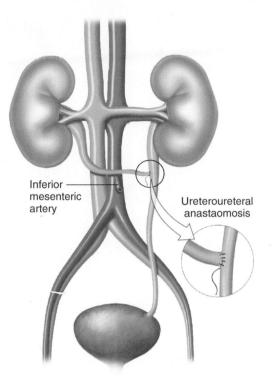

Figure 5.14 Transureteroureterostomy

Transureteroureterostomy (Fig. 5.14)

Alternatively, injuries involving the distal half of the ureter with insufficient bladder capacity or severe pelvic scarring can be managed by transureteroureterostomy. The posterior peritoneum is incised, exposing both ureters. The diseased ureter is brought carefully through a retroperitoneal window, avoiding any angulation. A 1.5-cm longitudinal ureterotomy is made on the medial surface of the recipient ureter, and an end-to-side anastomosis is created with interrupted fine absorbable sutures. The donor ureter should course above

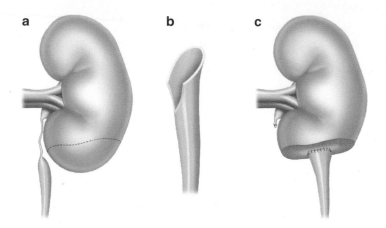

FIGURE 5.15 Ureterocalycostomy. (**a**) Amputated inferior renal pole. (**b**) Wide ureteral spatulation. (**c**) Completed ureterocalyceal anastomosis

the inferior mesenteric artery to avoid inadvertent ureteral impingement. This procedure can potentially jeopardize the integrity of the normal ureter and should be used selectively.

Ureterocalycostomy (Fig. 5.15)

An ureterocalycostomy can be used for extensive injuries to the ureteropelvic junction and proximal ureter. The lower pole of the involved kidney is amputated, exposing the infundibulum of the inferior calyx. The ureter is generously spatulated, allowing for a direct end-to-end ureterocalyceal anastomosis. This procedure involves excessive renal dissection and is fraught with a high incidence of anastomotic stricture.

Complete Ureteral Injuries

For complete ureteral avulsions, a segment of ileum may be interposed as a ureteral substitute (Fig. 5.16). This cannot be done acutely because it requires a standard mechanical bowel prep. Moreover, it should not be used in patients with significant renal insufficiency (serum creatinine >2.0 mg/dl) in order to limit metabolic complications (i.e., hyperchloremic

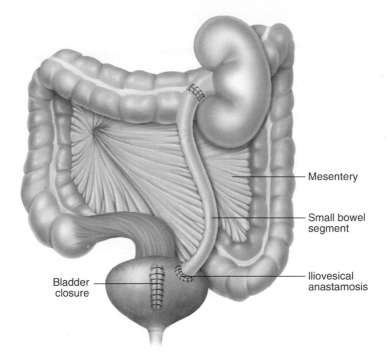

Mesentery

Small bowel segment

Bladder closure

Iliovesical anastamosis

FIGURE 5.16 Complete ureteral replacement using an ileal interposition

acidosis from urinary absorption). Additional contraindications to ileal interposition include radiation enteritis, inflammatory bowel disease, and bladder dysfunction.

The procedure involves medial mobilization of the ipsilateral colon, ureteral identification, and isolation of a 20–25-cm segment of ileum, 15 cm proximal to the ileocecal junction. Bowel continuity is reestablished, and the ileal neoureter is positioned posteriorly in an isoperistaltic fashion. An end-to-end pyeloileal anastomosis is completed proximally, and an end-to-side ileovesical anastomosis fashioned distally, without tunneling.

In patients with a solitary kidney or significantly compromised renal function, complete ureteral avulsions can be managed by renal autotransplantation. The affected kidney is transplanted into the iliac fossa with vascular anastomoses of the renal and iliac vessels. Urinary continuity is restored by means of a pyelovesicostomy.

Drainage

- All ureteral injuries should be stented to maximize urinary diversion. An internal double-J stent can be used for this purpose. The ureteral stent is usually maintained for 2–6 weeks, depending on the extent of ureteral repair.
- A retroperitoneal drain should be placed at the site of the reconstruction to limit urinoma formation. The retroperitoneal drain is maintained for at least 48 h or until any urinary leakage subsides.
- The bladder should be decompressed using a transurethral or suprapubic catheter, alone or in combination. The bladder catheter is usually removed within a week, although it may need to remain longer to avoid ureteral reflux.

Complications

Complications of ureteral injuries include:
- Prolonged urinary extravasation
- Infection
- Urinoma
- Fistula (including vesicovaginal and ureterovaginal)
- Stricture
- Progressive renal failure with acidosis and upper urinary tract decompensation

Outcome

A delay in diagnosis is the most important contributory factor in morbidity related to ureteral injury. A high index of suspicion must be maintained to obtain a satisfactory outcome in these usually polytraumatized patients.

Pelvic Fractures and Injuries to the Urinary System

Etiology

Pelvic trauma can be divided by mechanism into two groups, low energy and high energy, based on the energy exchanged in the impact.

Low-energy pelvic fractures most commonly occur from domestic falls, sports injuries, or low-velocity vehicular accidents. They usually result in isolated fractures of the pelvic ring without damaging the integrity of the pelvic structures. Approximately one-third of all pelvic fractures are low energy.

High-energy pelvic fractures are usually a consequence of motor vehicle and motorcycle accidents, pedestrian injuries, or falls from heights >4 m. They often result in multiple injuries to the pelvic ring, including fractures of the pubic rami, iliac wings, and sacrum, displacement of the pubic rami, and disruption of the sacroiliac joint. Associated injuries with high-energy pelvic fractures are listed in Table 5.6 (Demetriades et al. 2002).

TABLE 5.6 Associated injuries with high-energy pelvic fractures

Extremity fractures
Tibia
Femur
Central nervous system
Head
Spine
Chest
Abdomen
Liver
Lower urinary tract (bladder and urethra)
Spleen
Diaphragm
Bowel

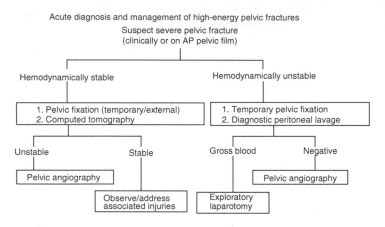

FIGURE 5.17 Algorithm for the acute diagnosis and management of high-energy pelvic fractures

Diagnosis (Fig. 5.17)

The accurate assessment of a patient with a suspected pelvic fracture depends not only on the traditional history, physical, laboratory, and radiographic examination but also on available details of the mechanism of injury (including the type, direction, and magnitude of the force involved). In a traumatized patient, visual signs suggestive of a pelvic fracture include abnormal leg length, rotational lower extremity deformities, and open perineal wounds.

Initial Evaluation

- The initial evaluation of any patient suspected of having a pelvic fracture should include a *gentle* manual examination of the pelvic ring for vertical and rotational instability. In an alert patient, pain on palpation of the pelvic ring is an important finding. In an unconscious patient, *gentle* anteroposterior and lateral-medial pelvic compression can be used to evaluate stability. Repeated examinations should be avoided as they can potentiate bleeding.

- Examination of the abdomen often demonstrates voluntary guarding with suprapubic dullness to percussion.
- The flank, scrotum, and perineum should be inspected for the presence of swelling or hematoma.
- A digital rectal exam should be performed on all patients, and a vaginal examination in all females to identify concomitant injuries. The presence of rectal or vaginal blood suggests injury to these organs.
- Meatal bleeding signifies a posterior urethral injury and should preclude transurethral catheterization.
- A complete blood count and appropriate vital signs can be used to estimate the degree of blood loss.
- Radiographs of the cervical spine, chest, abdomen, anteroposterior pelvis and extremities should be performed on all high-energy pelvic fractures; imaging of low-energy fractures can be confined to the pelvis.

Hemodynamically Unstable Patients

- In hemodynamically *un*stable patients, the primary goal is to identify and control bleeding.
- The pelvis should be stabilized using either a proprietary device or simply a bedsheet as a binder. This maneuver decreases pelvic volume, stabilizes the fracture, and potentially limits venous bleeding. Military antishock trousers (MAST) can also be used to limit further blood loss by increasing blood return from the lower extremities to the central circulation.
- Thoracic and abdominal sources of bleeding must be excluded. Chest radiographs suffice to rule out significant thoracic bleeding. Peritoneal lavage is used to assess intra-abdominal bleeding. This is performed preferably using a supraumbilical open technique. False-positive results can occur from contamination by the pelvic hematoma. In order to limit false readings, a positive aspiration is considered when *gross* rather than microscopic blood is obtained. Although a negative lavage is accurate in ruling out an intraperitoneal injury, it can miss a retroperitoneal injury.

- Alternatively, focused abdominal ultrasonography can be used for the initial evaluation of the intra-abdominal organs. The results of these tests are essential in triaging unstable patients between the operating room and the angiography suite.

A patient who is hemodynamically unstable should not be taken for CT imaging.

Hemodynamically Stable Patients

In hemodynamically stable patients, additional radiographs should be obtained to identify and classify all injuries; this is preferably accomplished using CT scans of the pelvis and abdomen.

Lower Urinary Tract Injuries

Approximately 10–12 % of high-energy pelvic fractures will result in lower urinary tract injuries. Blunt bladder ruptures and posterior urethral disruptions occur almost exclusively with pelvic fractures. There is a loose association between the type of pelvic fracture and the likelihood of a lower urinary tract injury. In general, injuries to the anterior pelvic arch have a higher likelihood of a concomitant lower urinary tract injury (Koraitim et al. 1966).

A delay in diagnosing a concomitant lower urinary tract injury has been reported in approximately 20 % of patients (Ziran et al. 2005). Common causes of missed diagnosis include failure to suspect an injury and misinterpretation of imaging studies.

Bladder Injuries

- 60 % of pelvic fracture-associated bladder ruptures are extraperitoneal, 30 % are intraperitoneal, and 10 % have both an intra- and extraperitoneal component.
- Most bladder ruptures are from a burst rather than a laceration injury, suggesting that it is the strong external force applied to the pelvis rather than a direct perforation by a bony spicule that disrupts the bladder.

Posterior Urethral Injuries

- Posterior urethral disruptions result from the severe shearing forces needed to fracture the pelvis being transmitted to the weakest portion of the urethra—the bulbomembranous junction.

Bladder Neck and Prostatic Injuries

- Injuries to the bladder neck and prostatic urethra are more common in children.

Classification

Although several classifications of pelvic fractures have been proposed, the most comprehensive is the Young system. It is based on the type and direction of the injurious force applied to the pelvic ring. The injuries are classified as follows:

Lateral Compression Injuries

Lateral compression injuries: transverse fracture of pubic rami, ipsilateral, or contralateral to posterior injury.

Type I: sacral compression on side of impact
Type II: crescent (iliac wing) fracture on side of impact
Type III: Type I or II injuries on side of impact; contralateral open-book (anteroposterior compression) injury

Lateral compression injuries occur from a laterally applied force and result in stretching rather than tearing of the pelvic ligaments. They are usually not associated with significant pelvic hemorrhage but often have associated injuries (e.g., intraperitoneal, pulmonary, or head).

Anteroposterior Compression Injuries

Anteroposterior compression injuries: symphyseal diastasis and/or longitudinal rami fracture.

Type I: slight widening of pubic symphysis and/or anterior sacroiliac (SI) joint; stretched but intact anterior SI, sacrotuberous, and sacrospinous ligaments; intact posterior SI ligaments

Type II: widened anterior SI joint; disrupted anterior SI, sacrotuberous, and sacrospinous ligaments; intact posterior SI ligaments

Type III: complete SI joint disruption with lateral displacement; disrupted anterior SI, sacrotuberous, and sacrospinous ligaments; disrupted posterior SI ligaments

Anteroposterior compression injuries result from forces applied to the anterior or posterior superior iliac spine areas, either directly or indirectly, via the lower extremities or ischial tuberosities. They result in pelvic ligament tears, open symphysis and sacroiliac joints, and significant bleeding.

Vertical Shear Injuries

Vertical shear injuries: symphyseal diastasis or vertical displacement anteriorly and posteriorly, usually through the SI joint, occasionally through the iliac wing and/or sacrum.

Vertical shear injuries occur when the pelvis is stressed vertically or longitudinally. The classic mechanism is a fall from a height, landing on an extended lower extremity. In addition, these injuries can occur when a victim is struck from above (by a falling object) or by forces applied to the pelvis from an extended lower extremity during a motor vehicle accident (by leg extension against the floorboard just prior to impact). Such injuries result in significant trauma to the pelvic ligaments.

Combined Mechanical Injuries

Combined mechanical injuries: combination of other injury patterns (most commonly lateral compression and vertical shear injuries).

Management

Low-Energy Pelvic Fractures

Low-energy pelvic fractures usually can be managed nonoperatively with gentle mobilization and protected weight bearing. Prolonged bed rest, pelvic suspension, and body casts are not advised.

High-Energy Pelvic Fractures (Fig. 5.17)

Treatment of high-energy pelvic fractures depends on the patients overall condition, associated injuries, and the specifics of the pelvic disruption.

- As outlined earlier, pelvic stabilization should be performed promptly to limit further bleeding. This can be accomplished immediately with a temporary device or within the first 4 h after the injury (once the patient is hemodynamically stable) with an external fixator. The external fixator can be easily applied in the resuscitation suite and may be all that is required to stabilize the fracture. Its limitation is that it allows reduction of only anterior and not posterior pelvic ring disruptions.
- If despite these maneuvers hemodynamic instability persists, patients with a positive peritoneal lavage should undergo exploratory laparotomy, and those with a negative lavage should be taken for pelvic angiography with attempt at selective angioembolization.
- Once the patient has been effectively hemodynamically stabilized and all associated injuries addressed, definitive management of the pelvic fracture can be accomplished using internal fixation. This is usually deferred for several days to allow resolution of the retroperitoneal bleeding. Internal fixation is performed in the operating room using a variety of techniques depending on the pelvic fracture pattern.

Lower Urinary Tract Injuries

In general, lower urinary tract injuries should be addressed after the initial resuscitation when the patient is stabilized. The appropriate management of associated injuries to the bladder and posterior urethra are covered in their respective chapters. Injuries involving the bladder neck and/or prostatic urethra require prompt surgical repair to avoid incontinence.

Complications

- Long-term pain disability
- Infection
- Thromboembolism
- Sexual dysfunction
- Urinary and/or bowel incontinence

Outcome

Pelvic fractures are severe injuries that are associated with a high incidence of morbidity and mortality. Prompt identification and control of pelvic hemorrhage is pivotal in decreasing pelvic fracture-related complications. Identification of associated organ injuries and appropriate treatment is paramount in achieving a successful outcome. The possibility of a lower urinary tract injury should always be considered in patients presenting with high-energy pelvic fractures.

Bladder Injuries

Etiology

The bladder is second to the kidneys in frequency of injury, accounting for approximately 25 % of all civilian genitourinary injuries.

External Trauma

External bladder injuries are caused by either blunt or penetrating trauma to the lower abdomen, pelvis, or perineum.

Blunt trauma is the more common mechanism, usually by a sudden deceleration such as a high-speed motor vehicle accident or fall or from an external blow to the lower abdomen. More than 95 % of blunt bladder ruptures occur with pelvic fractures. Other associated injuries include long bone fractures and central nervous system and chest injuries. Overall, approximately 10 % of high-energy pelvic fractures result in bladder rupture. Although with a pelvic fracture a spicule of bone can lacerate the bladder, more commonly it is the strong shearing or bursting force exerted on the pelvic ring that tears the bladder.

Penetrating trauma accounts for approximately 25 % of external bladder injuries in North America and is most commonly a result of gunshot wounds. Stab wounds and spike impalements are less frequent causes. More than half of the penetrating bladder traumas have associated bowel injuries.

Iatrogenic Trauma
(Armenakas et al. 2004; Dobrowolski et al. 2002)

The bladder is the most frequently injured organ during pelvic surgery. Predisposing factors include scarring from prior

TABLE 5.7 Causes of iatrogenic bladder injuries

Transurethral surgery

   Transurethral resection of bladder tumor (TURBt)

   Transurethral resection of prostate (TURP)

   Cystolithotripsy or cystolitholapaxy

Gynecologic surgery

   Abdominal or vaginal hysterectomy

   Cesarean section

   Pelvic mass excision

   Transvaginal surgery for prolapse and incontinence

Abdominal surgery

   Colon resection (for malignancy, diverticulitis, or inflammatory
   bowel disease)

Laparoscopic abdominal or pelvic surgery

surgery or radiation, inflammation, and extensive tumor burden. Common causes of iatrogenic bladder injuries are listed in Table 5.7.

Diagnosis

A bladder injury should be suspected after any external lower abdominal or pelvic trauma or surgery in this region.

History

Patients commonly complain of pelvic or lower abdominal pain and distention and may be unable to urinate.

Clinical Findings

External Trauma

The physical examination should include carefully performed pelvic and rectal examinations to identify concomitant injuries. External injuries from a blunt mechanism often present with hemodynamic instability because of extensive pelvic hemorrhage from the associated pelvic fracture.

Iatrogenic Trauma

Most iatrogenic bladder injuries are identified intraoperatively. Frequent findings include:

- Urinary extravasation
- Visible laceration
- Appearance of a Foley catheter in the operative field
- Gas distention of the urinary drainage bag (during laparoscopy)

In cases of a delay in diagnosis, patients may present with abdominal distention, ileus, urinary leakage from the incision, and anuria.

Laboratory Tests

The hallmark of a bladder injury is hematuria. Gross hematuria occurs in at least 95 % of bladder ruptures from blunt injury; the remainder have microscopic hematuria. In contrast, approximately one-half of patients with penetrating bladder injuries present with gross hematuria. With delayed recognition, serum levels of blood urea nitrogen (BUN) and creatinine may be elevated due to transperitoneal urinary absorption.

Imaging
(Gomez et al. 2004)

- Cystography is the most accurate imaging test for diagnosing a bladder injury.
- Prior to catheterization, the urethral meatus must be inspected. Blood at the meatus is a contraindication to urethral catheterization in the setting of pelvic trauma as it strongly suggests a urethral injury which requires confirmation by retrograde urethrography.

- Either conventional or CT cystography can be used with equivalent accuracy. In each case, the bladder must be filled in a *retrograde* manner with at least 350 ml of contrast. The cystogram phase of a CT, with intravenous contrast alone, is inaccurate in diagnosing a bladder injury.
- With CT cystography, the contrast should be diluted (approximately 5:1) to avoid a "whiteout" effect which can obscure visualization. Post-drainage films should be obtained only with conventional cystography since a posterior leak may be obscured by the contrast-filled bladder.
- The amount of contrast extravasation cannot be used to determine the extent of bladder injury as this is dependent on the rate and volume of contrast infused.
- Most iatrogenic bladder injuries are diagnosed intraoperatively without bladder imaging.

Indications for Imaging (Morey et al. 2001) (Fig. 5.18)

Indications for radiographic bladder imaging include:

- Any *penetrating* injury to the lower abdomen or pelvis
- Any *blunt* injury presenting with either of the following:
    - Gross hematuria
    - Microscopic hematuria and a pelvic fracture
    - Any clinical suspicion of a bladder injury (e.g., suprapubic tenderness, inability to void, or altered sensorium)
- Any suspicion of an iatrogenic bladder injury during or after abdominal or pelvic surgery

Imaging Findings

Radiographic findings of bladder injuries include contusions and extra- and intraperitoneal ruptures. They are differentiated by the presence or absence of contrast extravasation and its pattern.

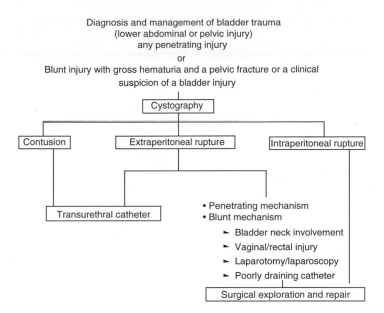

Figure 5.18 Algorithm for the diagnosis and management of bladder injuries

Contusions (Fig. 5.19)

Contusions are injuries to the bladder wall without loss of continuity. The bladder is typically teardrop shaped because of external compression from a large pelvic hematoma. There is no extravasation of contrast.

Extraperitoneal Ruptures (Fig. 5.20)

Extraperitoneal bladder ruptures are characterized by starburst contrast extravasation usually limited to the true pelvis. However, the extravasation may extend through the obturator foramen and inguinal canal to the thigh and scrotum inferiorly and superiorly within the retroperitoneal space. Inferior extravasation of contrast suggests the possibility of bladder neck or prostatic involvement by direct extension of the laceration. Fluoroscopy may be helpful in better identifying the pattern of extravasation in such cases.

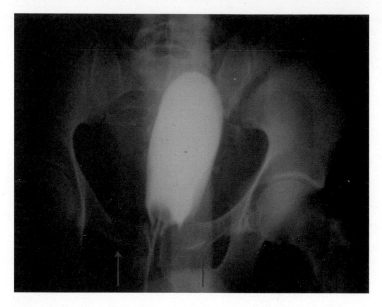

FIGURE 5.19 Teardrop-shaped bladder consistent with a contusion. Bilateral pubic rami fractures are shown with the *arrows*

Intraperitoneal Ruptures (Fig. 5.21)

Intraperitoneal bladder ruptures are distinguished by extravasation of contrast which outlines loops of bowel.

Injury Classification

Bladder injuries are classified based on the extent of injury, as follows:

Grade I: contusion, intramural hematoma, or partial-thickness laceration

Grade II: extraperitoneal bladder wall laceration <2 cm

Grade III: extraperitoneal bladder wall laceration >2 cm or intraperitoneal bladder wall laceration <2 cm

Grade IV: intraperitoneal bladder wall laceration >2 cm

Grade V: intraperitoneal or extraperitoneal bladder wall laceration extending into bladder neck or ureteral orifice (trigone)

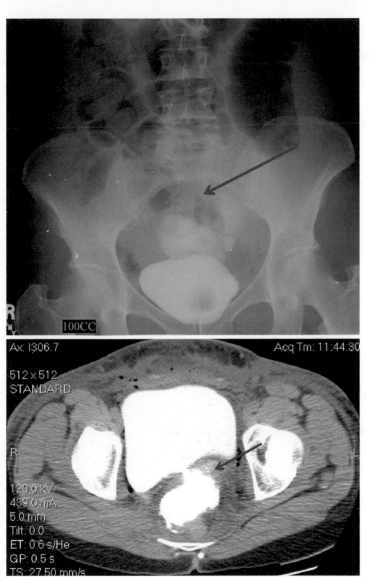

FIGURE 5.20 Conventional and CT cystograms showing an extraperitoneal bladder rupture (*arrows*) in the same patient

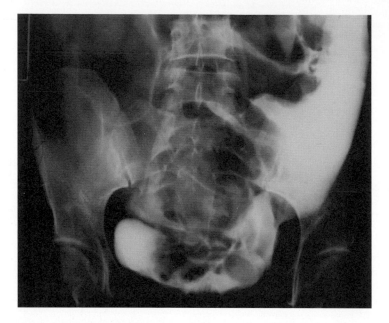

FIGURE 5.21 Intraperitoneal bladder rupture depicted by contrast outlining loops of bowel

Management
(Gomez et al. 2004) (Fig. 5.18)

Management of a bladder injury depends on the overall status of the patient, the grade of injury, and the extent of any associated injuries.

Bladder Contusions and Hematomas

Bladder contusions and hematomas can be treated by transurethral catheter drainage alone. This is maintained until the hematuria visibly resolves.

TABLE 5.8 Indications for surgical repair of extraperitoneal bladder ruptures

Bladder neck or prostatic extension

Concomitant vaginal or rectal injury

Laparotomy for associated injury

Iatrogenic injury identified during laparotomy

Failure of adequate catheter drainage

Extraperitoneal Ruptures (Fig. 5.18)

Most extraperitoneal bladder ruptures usually can be managed nonoperatively provided there is good catheter drainage and no infection. If the catheter does not drain properly or if the patient is going to the operating room for repair of other injuries (such as pelvic fixation), formal surgical bladder repair is advised. Additional indications for surgical repair of extraperitoneal bladder ruptures are listed in Table 5.8. Any one of these findings requires an operative approach.

Intraperitoneal Ruptures

Intraperitoneal bladder ruptures are usually large stellate lacerations at the bladder dome and require immediate surgical exploration

Bladder Exploration and Reconstruction (Fig. 5.22)

- The bladder is explored through a midline infraumbilical incision, avoiding dissection of the pelvic hematoma.
- A peritoneotomy is made, allowing inspection of the abdominal viscera.
- General principles of bladder reconstruction include:
  - Inspection of the bladder neck and orifices
  - Limited debridement of nonviable tissue

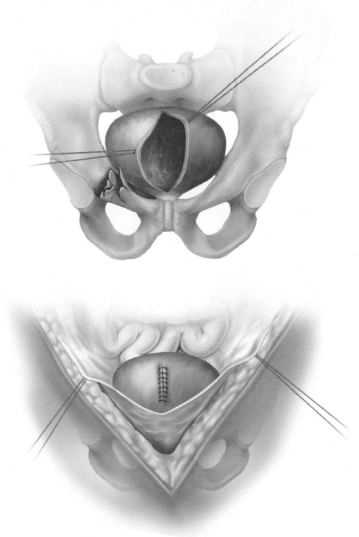

FIGURE 5.22 Bladder exploration through an anterior midline cystotomy, avoiding dissection of the pelvic hematoma

- Suturing of the laceration preferably from within the bladder
- Appropriate bladder drainage

- The bladder is closed in two layers using absorbable sutures.
- In males, both suprapubic and transurethral catheters are preferred; in females, a transurethral Foley catheter suffices.
- Catheter drainage is maintained for 7–10 days at which time a cystogram is performed to ensure adequate healing.

Complications

Early

- Persistent hematuria
- Uroascites
- Infection
- Sepsis

Late

- Bladder instability
- Incontinence
- Fistula
- Pseudodiverticulum

Outcome

Mortality in patients with external bladder trauma approaches 20 % and results from the associated injuries rather than the bladder laceration. Iatrogenic injuries are usually diagnosed and repaired promptly, limiting sequelae from delayed identification.

Posterior Urethral Injuries

Etiology

External Trauma

Injuries to the posterior urethra from external trauma occur almost exclusively with pelvic fractures. Specifically, with a compression or deceleration-impact injury, the severe shearing forces necessary to fracture the pelvis are transmitted to the bulbomembranous junction, the weakest portion of the urethra, resulting in its disruption. The usual mechanism is a motor vehicle-, pedestrian-, or work-related accident. Overall, the male posterior urethra is injured in up to 6 % of all pelvic fractures. Most patients have multiple associated organ injuries, including to the abdomen, chest, head, and long bones.

Iatrogenic Trauma

Surgical injuries can occur from various procedures on the prostate, including radical or simple prostatectomies, transurethral prostatic reductive surgeries, and radiation therapy. These usually involve the bladder neck region but can extend distally to involve the entire prostate and/or the external sphincter mechanism. The incidence of anastomotic stricture after radical prostatectomy ranges from 7 to 25 %, with the higher values corresponding to patients undergoing salvage surgery or adjuvant radiation therapy (Santucci and McAninch 2002).

Diagnosis

External Trauma

A posterior urethral injury should be suspected in any patient with a *pelvic fracture and blood at the meatus*.

Other signs and symptoms include hematuria, pain on urination, and inability to void. A high-riding prostate is an unreliable finding. All patients should have a rectal examination to evaluate for a concomitant bowel injury.

Iatrogenic Trauma

Iatrogenic injuries often manifest gradually with obstructive-type symptoms. Patients may accommodate to their declining voiding symptoms and delay in seeking medical attention.

Imaging

Any patient suspected of having a urethral injury should undergo dynamic retrograde urethrography before transurethral catheterization. The diagnosis of a posterior urethral injury from external trauma is made by retrograde urethrography (see section "Anterior Urethral Injuries"). Extravasation of contrast is diagnostic of a urethral disruption (Fig. 5.23).

In patients who experience posttraumatic erectile dysfunction, a baseline color penile duplex ultrasound can be used to assess penile vascular anatomy.

Cystoscopy

In contrast, most iatrogenic injuries are diagnosed cystoscopically. These injuries result in urethral narrowing with preservation of urethral continuity. Although a voiding cystourethrogram may be helpful in making the diagnosis, provided a catheter can be passed transurethrally, cystoscopic confirmation is almost always required.

Classification

See section "Anterior Urethral Injuries."

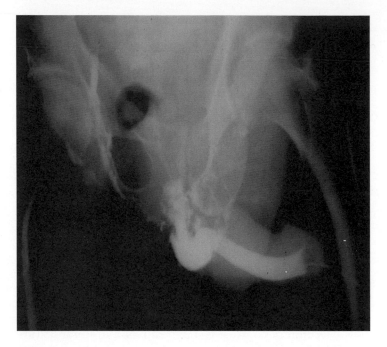

FIGURE 5.23 Retrograde urethrogram with extravasation of contrast consistent with a posterior urethral disruption

Initial Management

External Trauma (Fig. 5.24)

The initial approach to the management of posterior urethral disruptions depends on the patient's overall condition and the treating surgeon's expertise. Since most patients with pelvic fractures have significant coexisting trauma, immediate consideration should be given to resuscitative measures and treatment of the associated injuries.

The two options for managing posterior urethral disruptions initially are (Husmann et al. 1990; Mouravier et al. 2005):

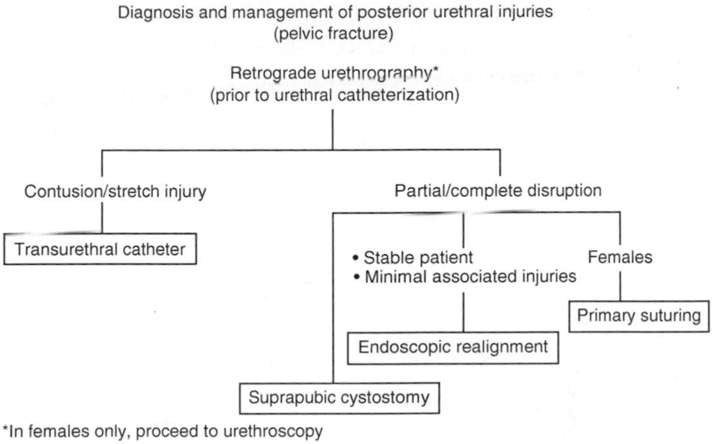

Diagnosis and management of posterior urethral injuries
(pelvic fracture)

Retrograde urethrography*
(prior to urethral catheterization)

Contusion/stretch injury

Transurethral catheter

Partial/complete disruption

• Stable patient
• Minimal associated injuries

Females

Primary suturing

Endoscopic realignment

Suprapubic cystostomy

*In females only, proceed to urethroscopy

FIGURE 5.24 Algorithm for the diagnosis and management of posterior urethral disruptions

- Suprapubic cystostomy with delayed urethral reconstruction
- Endoscopic realignment
  - *The easiest, safest, and most readily available initial management option for any posterior urethral disruption is the placement of a suprapubic cystostomy tube.* This is preferably done using an open approach to identify and repair coexisting bladder injuries. After the patient has adequately recovered from the associated injuries and the urethral injury has stabilized, the urethra can be evaluated radiographically and the appropriate reconstructive procedure planned.
  - Alternatively, endoscopic realignment can be attempted in order to decrease the likelihood of subsequent stricture formation and need for delayed open urethral reconstruction.
  - Immediate suture repair of a posterior urethral injury is contraindicated. Such intervention exposes the polytraumatized patient to unnecessary risks and is fraught with an unacceptably high complication rate.

- Approximately 15 % of patients with posterior urethral disruptions have an associated bladder rupture. The bladder must be evaluated surgically (during placement of an open cystostomy tube) or cystographically (after placement of a percutaneous cystostomy tube).
- As with anterior urethral injuries, posterior urethral contusions and stretch injuries can be managed with transurethral catheterization.

Iatrogenic Trauma

- Treatment depends on the etiology and extent of scarring.
- Options include (Santucci and McAninch 2002; Wessells et al. 1998):

  - *Urethral dilation,* which is palliative but may suffice in achieving a satisfactory outcome in select patients.
  - *Endoscopic treatments,* including internal urethrotomy and transurethral resection or lasering of scar tissue.
  - *Open repair,* preferably by anastomotic urethroplasty.

Minimally Invasive Techniques

Open Suprapubic Cystostomy

- The bladder is exposed through a midline incision.
- The entire bladder is inspected from within, avoiding any external dissection which may disrupt the pelvic hematoma.
- Any bladder lacerations are repaired in two layers with absorbable sutures.
- The bladder neck and ureteral orifices should be inspected.
- A large suprapubic catheter (22Fr) is placed in the bladder prior to closure.

Percutaneous Suprapubic Cystostomy

This can be performed in the resuscitation suite, preferably using sonographic guidance.

- A 16-Fr percutaneous tube should be used to permit adequate urinary drainage.
- A cystogram is done to exclude an associated bladder injury which should be identified and repaired promptly.

Endoscopic Realignment (Fig. 5.25)

This may be considered in patients with minimal associated organ injuries. Situations where endoscopic realignment may be beneficial include:

- Concomitant bladder rupture
- During open reduction and internal fixation of the pelvic ring
- Associated rectal and bladder injuries
- Severe bladder displacement

Many endoscopic techniques have been described to bridge the urethral distraction defect including the use of

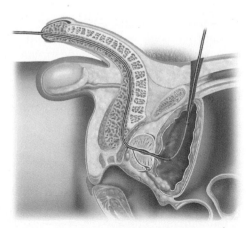

FIGURE 5.25 Endoscopic realignment of the posterior urethra using a retrograde and antegrade approach

interlocking and magnetic sounds. Basically, a catheter should be passed antegrade through the bladder neck under direct vision. If this is successfully advanced to the urethral meatus, a second catheter is tied to this and advanced retrograde into the bladder. Flexible cystoscopy may be helpful in identifying the proper course. Dissection of the bladder neck and prostate are discouraged, and traction should never be used. If urethral continuity cannot be reestablished, the procedure should be aborted and urinary diversion accomplished via a suprapubic catheter.

The advantage of endoscopic realignment is the potential avoidance of a subsequent urethral reconstruction. Although approximately 50 % of posterior urethral injuries treated this way may not require an open repair, often multiple endoscopic procedures are needed to manage the ensuing stricture. Limitations of endoscopic realignment include difficulty in positioning patients because of their pelvic fractures and anesthetic complications from additional surgery.

Definitive Management

Urethral Reconstruction
(Webster and Ramon 1991; Kizer et al. 2007)

Reconstruction of the posterior urethra should be delayed for approximately 8–12 weeks or until the patient has healed from any significant associated organ injuries. The goals of open posterior urethral reconstruction include:

- Excision of scar tissue
- Creation of a direct urethral-urethral anastomosis
- Construction of an unobstructed urethral conduit

The procedure is performed as follows:

- The patient is placed in an exaggerated lithotomy position.
- A vertical perineal incision is made and carried down through the bulbocavernosus muscles, exposing the proximal bulbar urethra.

- The corpus spongiosum is mobilized circumferentially at this level, and the urethra is transected.
- A sound is passed via the suprapubic tract through the bladder neck to the point of obliteration.
- The sound is palpated within the scar tissue at the level of the urethral detachment, and the fibrotic tissue is sequentially excised to normal appearing urethral epithelium. Stay sutures are placed to facilitate identification of the normal proximal urethral lumen.
- The anterior urethra is then dissected distally off the ventral corporal bodies and mobilized caudally. If this maneuver is not sufficient in obtaining adequate urethral length for an uncompromised anastomosis, the following additional steps can be used to shorten the distance:

  - Midline separation of the corpora cavernosa
  - Inferior pubectomy
  - Rerouting of the spongiosum below the left corpora cavernosa.

- A direct anastomosis of the bulbar urethra to the prostatic urethral apex is done over an 18-Fr Foley catheter, using interrupted 5–0 absorbable sutures. A single layer is used dorsally, incorporating the urethral mucosa and spongiosum, whereas a two-layer closure is used ventrally, approximating the urethral mucosa and spongiosum as separate layers.
- The perineal incision is closed in several layers with absorbable sutures (Fig. 5.26).

In rare instances, a transpubic approach may be used in order to improve visualization of the prostatomembranous regions (such as with severe posterior urethral displacement or multiple fistulous tracts). It is accomplished through a separate lower abdominal incision extending to the base of the penis. A wedge of pubis is removed with a Gigli saw. Orthopedic sequelae of pubic resection are negligible because the anterior two-thirds of the pelvic ring is non-weight-bearing.

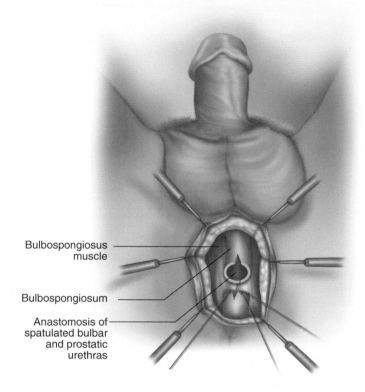

Bulbospongiosus
muscle

Bulbospongiosum

Anastomosis of
spatulated bulbar
and prostatic
urethras

FIGURE 5.26 Anastomotic bulboprostatic urethroplasty

Female Urethral Injuries
(Venn et al. 1999; Perry and Husmann 1992)

Female urethral injuries from external trauma are uncommon. Approximately 4 % of significant pelvic fractures will have an associated urethral injury. Iatrogenic injuries can occur during transvaginal procedures, such as pubovaginal slings, and cystocele repairs.

A urethral injury should be suspected in any patient with a *pelvic fracture and blood at the vaginal introitus*. A careful pelvic examination should be performed in all cases. Often, a vaginal laceration may be the only clinical indicator of a urethral injury. Additional findings may include labial swelling or ecchymosis, hematuria, and rectal tears. Concomitant bladder injuries occur in up to 70 % of patients.

Female urethral injuries are best evaluated cystoscopically. Urethrography is technically difficult because of limitations in adequately occluding the urethral meatus during retrograde injection of contrast which leads to extravasation and poor visualization.

Injuries can range from lacerations to complete avulsions. In all cases, prompt identification and primary surgical repair are paramount in limiting complications, including incontinence and urethrovaginal fistula formation.

Complications

Complications of posterior urethral injuries include urinary retention, incontinence, erectile dysfunction, urethral stricture and urethrocutaneous fistula. Incontinence and erectile dysfunction are a consequence of the initial pelvic neurovascular injury rather than the surgical management.

Outcome

Posterior urethral injures can result in devastating long-term consequences. To a young person, the potential complications of erectile dysfunction, stricture, and incontinence often create lifelong morbidity. Management of these injuries can be complex and depends on the individual case and the surgeon's expertise. As a general rule, initial suprapubic cystostomy is the simplest option. Alternatively, endoscopic realignment can be attempted. The advantage to this latter procedure is its lower subsequent stricture rate (approximately 50 % vs. 95 %). Contemporary series suggest similar erectile dysfunction and incontinence rates of 30 and 10 %, respectively, for both procedures.

Disruption of the female urethra requires immediate surgical repair. Prompt urethral and bladder neck reconstruction are necessary to avoid posttraumatic incontinence.

Anterior Urethral Injuries

The anterior urethra is a 15-cm canal extending from the termination of the membranous urethra to the external meatus. Its function, in conjunction with the posterior urethra, is to serve as a conduit for the passage of urine and semen.

The anatomic subdivisions of the urethra are shown in Fig. 5.27.

Etiology

Iatrogenic Trauma

Iatrogenic urethral injuries are the most frequent causes of anterior urethral trauma. Examples of acute injuries include inadvertent Foley catheter balloon inflation in the urethra and traumatic lower urinary tract endoscopy (cystoscopy, transurethral surgery). These injuries are often minor and tend to be underreported. Chronic injuries occur primarily with indwelling catheters. The mechanism

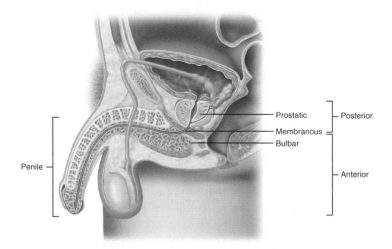

Figure 5.27 Anatomic subdivisions of the urethra

of injury includes necrosis from direct pressure or persistent inflammation from infection. These injuries may be unrecognized until they have progressed, resulting in urinary extravasation, abscess formation, and even fasciocutaneous tissue necrosis.

Blunt Trauma

Blunt mechanisms are the most common cause of acute anterior urethral injuries from external trauma. These include falls, blows to the perineum, and motor vehicle accidents. They are usually straddle injuries, causing forceful contact of the perineum with a blunt object such as bicycle handlebars or the top of a fence (Fig. 5.28). The bulbar urethral segment is most frequently involved.

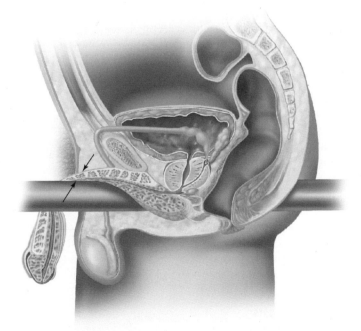

FIGURE 5.28 Straddle injury: a common mechanism of external blunt trauma to the anterior urethra

Penetrating

Penetrating injuries to the anterior urethra result predominantly from gunshot wounds. Often, these injuries occur in conjunction with penile or testicular trauma. Stab wounds rarely involve the urethra except when associated with genital self-mutilation.

Other less common causes of anterior urethral injuries include deliberate intraurethral insertion of foreign bodies, penile amputations, and penile ruptures (see section "Penile Injuries").

Diagnosis (Rosenstein and Alsikafi 2006)

History

The diagnosis of an acute urethral injury should be suspected from the history. A detailed voiding history should include the time of last urination, force of the urinary stream, painful urination, and hematuria.

Clinical Findings

Clinical findings suggestive of an anterior urethral injury include:
- *Blood at the meatus*
- Gross hematuria
- Pain on urination
- Inability to void
- Perineal and/or penile swelling or hematoma. The hematoma may extend superiorly to the abdomen and chest and inferiorly to the scrotum, perineum, and medial thighs (Fig. 5.29).
- Any penetrating injury to the penis or scrotum

Laboratory Tests

A urinalysis should be performed to assess the presence of hematuria.

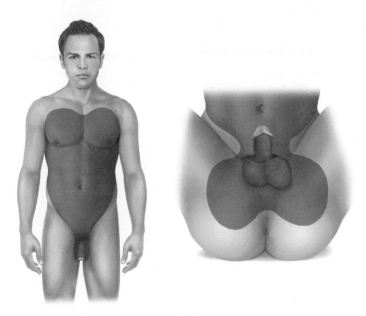

FIGURE 5.29 Extravasation of urine and/or blood with disruption of Buck's fascia can extend cranially beneath Scarpa's fascia (where it fuses with the coracoclavicular fascia) and caudally beneath Colle's fascia to the medial thighs (where it fuses with the fascia lata)

Imaging

Any patient with a history suggestive of a urethral injury or any clinical indicator of urethral trauma should undergo dynamic retrograde urethrography before any attempt is made at transurethral catheterization. The patients should be placed in a 30–45° oblique position with the lower thigh flexed 90° and the upper thigh straight (Fig. 5.30). A 12-Fr Foley catheter is placed into the fossa navicularis, and its balloon inflated to 2 cc to prevent reflux of contrast. Approximately 20–30 ml of undiluted water-soluble contrast material is instilled into the urethra under fluoroscopic guidance; images are taken while injecting. Extravasation of contrast material is diagnostic of a urethral disruption. Absence of urethral extravasation, in the setting of a urethral injury, suggests a urethral contusion.

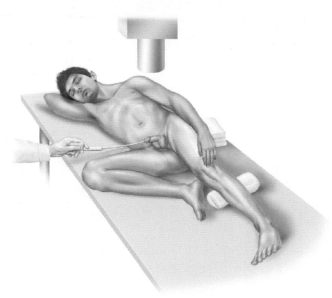

FIGURE 5.30 Retrograde urethrography performed with the patient in the oblique position. Contrast is instilled during fluoroscopy

Injury Classification

Urethral injuries are classified as follows:

Grade I: contusion: blood at the urethral meatus, normal urethrogram

Grade II: stretch injury: elongation of the urethra without extravasation on urethrography

Grade III: partial disruption: extravasation of contrast at injury site with contrast visualized in the bladder

Grade IV: complete disruption: extravasation of contrast at injury site without bladder visualization, <2 cm urethral separation

Grade V: complete disruption: complete transection with >2 cm urethral separation or extension in the prostate or vagina

Management
(McAninch 1981; Husmann et al. 1993) (Fig. 5.31)

The goal of initial treatment for any trauma to the urethra is avoidance of any maneuver that can potentiate the injury.

Urethral contusions and stretch injuries can be managed safely with transurethral catheterization maintained for 7–10 days.

Urethral disruptions are best managed with urinary diversion by means of a percutaneous suprapubic cystostomy. This is the easiest and safest option, applicable in all situations. Blind passage of a transurethral catheter is strongly discouraged.

- All complete blunt anterior urethral disruptions should be managed with cystotomy drainage, except those associated with penile ruptures.
- Select *partial* anterior urethral disruptions can be bridged using a flexible cystoscope to pass a guide wire followed by a council-tip catheter into the bladder. When attempted, this procedure should be done gently and aborted promptly

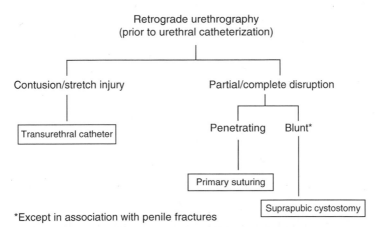

*Except in association with penile fractures

FIGURE 5.31 Algorithm for the diagnosis and management of anterior urethral injuries

if resistance or poor visualization is encountered. The disadvantage to this endoscopic realignment procedure is that it can potentiate the urethral injury by direct manipulation and/or extravasation of the irrigant.

- Penetrating urethral disruptions can be repaired primarily, providing that they are not associated with one or more of the following findings:

  - Hemodynamic instability
  - Multiple associated nongenital injuries
  - A large urethral defect requiring extensive reconstruction

Such cases should be managed with suprapubic urinary diversion.

- The cystostomy tube is maintained for at least 6 weeks at which time retrograde and voiding cystourethrograms are performed to identify the extent of injury. The appropriate reconstructive procedure can be scheduled, as needed, usually 8–12 weeks after the initial injury.

Anterior Urethral Reconstruction

- Immediate anterior urethral repair should be considered only in cases of penetrating urethral disruption, provided that they do not have any of the findings described earlier, and in any urethral injury associated with a penile rupture.
- Surgical repair of small mucosal tears can be accomplished with interrupted fine absorbable sutures, placed in a watertight fashion without compromising the urethral luminal size. An 18-Fr Foley catheter can be used to stent the repair.
- More extensive partial disruptions and select complete disruptions can be managed by primary excision and reanastomosis (Fig. 5.32).
- General principles of urethral reconstruction include:

  - Very minimal urethral debridement
  - Mobilization of the corpus spongiosum to obtain sufficient length for a tension-free anastomosis
  - Spatulation of both urethral ends on opposite sides

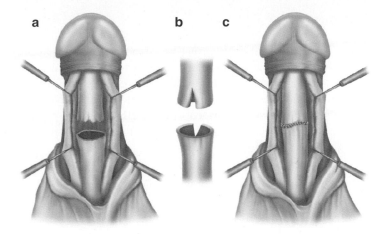

FIGURE 5.32 Anastomotic repair of an anterior urethral disruption.
(a) Conservative debridement. (b) Spatulation. (c) Reanastomosis

- Completion of a tension-free watertight urethral anastomosis over an 18-Fr Foley catheter using interrupted 5–0 absorbable sutures

- The urethral catheter is maintained for approximately 2 weeks after surgery. A voiding cystourethrogram is performed at the time of catheter removal to ensure complete healing.

If, at the time of initial exploration, the urethra is found to be so extensively disrupted that primary anastomosis is not feasible, either urethral marsupialization or suprapubic urinary diversion should be performed. Urethral replacement with grafts or flaps should be avoided in the acute trauma setting, as contamination or decreased blood supply can compromise such a repair.

Complications

Potential complications of anterior urethral injuries include stricture, infection, fistula, erectile dysfunction, and incontinence.

Outcome

An anterior urethral injury must be suspected in any patient after either blunt or penetrating trauma to the perineum or genitals or in anyone who has undergone recent transurethral instrumentation. Early diagnosis, prompt urinary diversion, and, where indicated, the appropriate urethral reconstruction are paramount in achieving a successful outcome with any anterior urethral injury.

Testicular Injuries

The anatomic characteristics of the testis protect it from injury. Its mobility and the strength of the tunica albuginea provide important safeguards from external trauma.

Etiology

- Most testicular injuries result from blunt trauma (80 %) and are usually unilateral. The most common causes are sport-related injuries, motor vehicle accidents, and assaults.
- Penetrating testicular injuries most frequently result from gunshots with one-third involving both testes. Most are associated with multiple injuries including to the thigh, penis, perincum, pelvis, urethra, and femoral vessels. Stab wounds involving the testes most often are self-inflicted during attempts at emasculation.

Diagnosis

Testicular injuries are diagnosed by history, physical examination, and sonography.

History

Typical complaints include intrascrotal pain and swelling after a direct blow or penetrating injury to the scrotum.

Clinical Findings (Fig. 5.33)

- Often, the exam is limited by patient discomfort, making it difficult to assess the extent of a testicular injury accurately by clinical means alone.
- In addition, the degree of injury may be out of proportion to the physical findings.

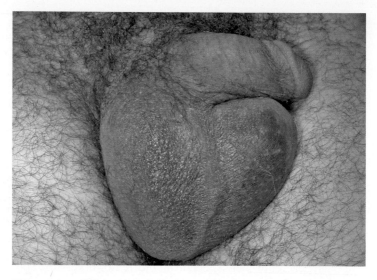

FIGURE 5.33 Clinical presentation: minimal scrotal ecchymosis and swelling

- On examination, the scrotum is usually discolored (ecchymotic), tender, and firm.
- Any penetrating injury to the scrotum suggests the likelihood of testicular involvement.

Imaging

- Because of the inconsistent clinical findings, the diagnosis of a blunt testicular injury should be confirmed by scrotal ultrasonography.
- A heterogeneous intratesticular echo pattern with loss of contour definition is the most consistent ultrasonographic finding of a testicular rupture (Buckley and McAninch 2006) (Fig. 5.34).
- Extruded testicular tissue or disruption of the tunica albuginea can be seen on occasion but is not a required sonographic criterion to confirm a rupture.

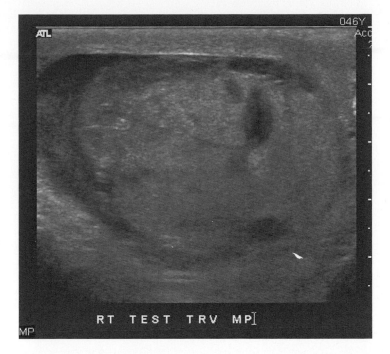

FIGURE 5.34 Scrotal ultrasonography of a blunt testicular rupture showing the heterogeneous parenchymal echo pattern

- Ultrasonography is not necessary for penetrating testicular trauma, as all such injuries require an operative approach.

Injury Classification

Testicular injuries are classified based on clinical and imaging information, as follows:

Grade I: contusion or hematoma

Grade II: subclinical laceration of tunica albuginea

Grade III: laceration of tunica albuginea with <50 % parenchymal loss

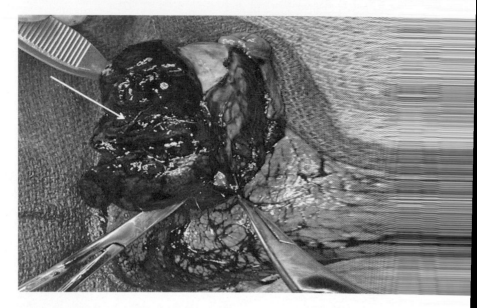

FIGURE 5.35 Ruptured testis with extensive seminife... extrusion (*arrow*)

Grade IV: major laceration of tunica albu...
             >50 % parenchymal loss
Grade V: total testicular destruction or avul...

Management

All penetrating testicular injuries and any blun... injury suggestive of a tunical disruption (clinical graphically) should be surgically explored and rep... testicular ruptures can be reconstructed primaril... and 5.36). Similarly, testicular gunshot wounds us... successful reconstructed. Stab wounds from self-e... have a low salvage rate because the spermatic c... transected (Phonsombat et al. 2008).

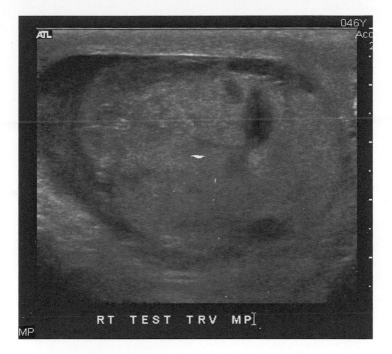

FIGURE 5.34 Scrotal ultrasonography of a blunt testicular rupture showing the heterogeneous parenchymal echo pattern

- Ultrasonography is not necessary for penetrating testicular trauma, as all such injuries require an operative approach.

Injury Classification

Testicular injuries are classified based on clinical and imaging information, as follows:

Grade I:	contusion or hematoma
Grade II:	subclinical laceration of tunica albuginea
Grade III:	laceration of tunica albuginea with <50 % parenchymal loss

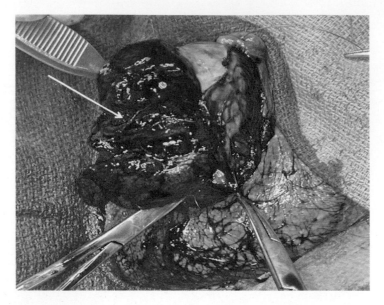

FIGURE 5.35 Ruptured testis with extensive seminiferous tubule extrusion (*arrow*)

Grade IV: major laceration of tunica albuginea with >50 % parenchymal loss

Grade V: total testicular destruction or avulsion

Management

All penetrating testicular injuries and any blunt testicular injury suggestive of a tunical disruption (clinically or sonographically) should be surgically explored and repaired. Most testicular ruptures can be reconstructed primarily (Figs. 5.35 and 5.36). Similarly, testicular gunshot wounds usually can be successful reconstructed. Stab wounds from self-emasculation have a low salvage rate because the spermatic cord is often transected (Phonsombat et al. 2008).

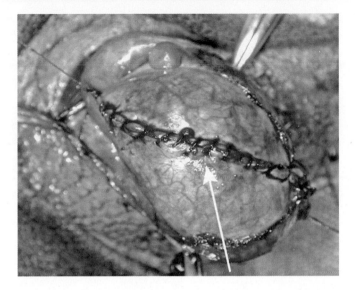

FIGURE 5.36 Completed testicular reconstruction. The *arrow* shows the sutured tunica albuginea

Testicular Exploration

- A transverse scrotal skin incision is used to expose the testis.
- General principles of testicular reconstruction include:
  - Complete exposure of the testis, epididymis and spermatic cord
  - Hematocele drainage
  - Judicious debridement of extruded seminiferous tubules with preservation of even marginal testicular tissue
  - Reapproximation of the tunica albuginea with absorbable sutures
  - Use of a tunica vaginalis graft for testicular coverage if the tunica albuginea is inadequate (Ferguson and Brandes 2007)

- For complete testicular destruction (usually a consequence of gunshot injuries), orchiectomy may be the only option.
- A small Penrose drain is placed which is usually removed after 24–48 h.
- The scrotum is closed in two layers, approximating the dartos fascia and skin, separately.

In cases of a delayed presentation, vascular integrity should be assessed with duplex ultrasonography and an orchiectomy performed if the testicle is felt to be necrotic.

Complications

Complications of testicular rupture include:

- Chronic pain
- Atrophy
- Impaired fertility
- Decreased social confidence

Outcome

With prompt diagnosis and exploration of testicular ruptures from a blunt or penetrating mechanism, a high testicular salvage rate can be achieved. A delay in operative management results in an orchiectomy rate approaching 50 % (Cass 1983). Although long-term effects of testicular trauma are not well defined due to insufficient follow-up, the limited available data suggests that endocrine function is preserved while seminal parameters may be compromised (Kudadia et al. 1996).

Penile Injuries

Penile injuries can occur from a variety of mechanisms. Their diagnosis is usually straightforward, but their management can be complicated by concomitant injuries and the need for both an acceptable functional and aesthetic result.

Etiology

The etiology of penile injuries is listed in Table 5.9.

- *Ruptures* (also referred to as fractures) occur in the erect penis, usually during intercourse or by abnormal bending during masturbation (Fig. 5.37a)
- *Amputations* (or mutilations) are usually self-inflicted or from an assault, or result from entrapment of clothes by heavy machinery.

TABLE 5.9 Etiology of penile injuries

Blunt
Ruptures
Penetrating
Amputations
Constrictions
Gunshot wounds
Stab wounds
Infections
Bites
Burns
Gangrene
Iatrogenic
Circumcision
Crush injuries/lacerations
Penile augmentation

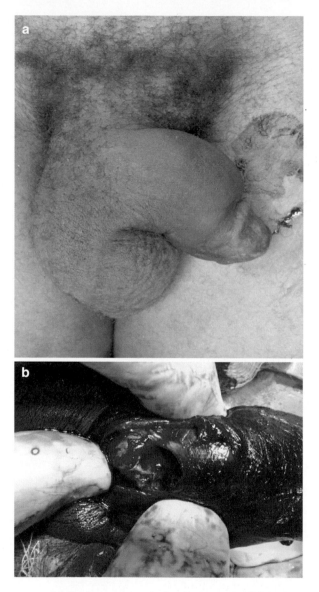

FIGURE 5.37 (a) Penile rupture during intercourse. (b) Defect in the tunica albuginea. (c) Simulated saline erection performed after completion of the repair

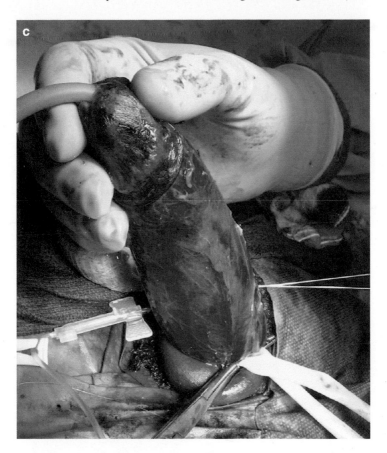

FIGURE 5.37 (continued)

- *Constrictions*, in adults, usually occur from penile rings used to enhance erections. In children, the injury is usually related to experimentation with strings, rubber bands, or hair.
- *Infections* result from bites, burns, or gangrene (necrotizing infections).
- *Gunshot and stab wounds*. Low-velocity gunshot wounds cause most penetrating penile injuries; up to 80 % are associated with other organ injuries, including the urethra, thigh, femoral vessels, pelvis, and perineum. Stab wounds are relatively infrequent.
- *Iatrogenic* injuries can occur from surgical procedures, such as circumcision, penile augmentation (Fig. 5.38), and

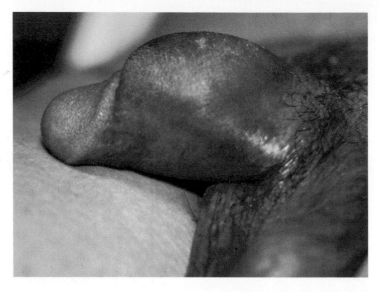

FIGURE 5.38 Iatrogenic penile deformity from penile augmentation using a dorsally placed AlloDerm graft

prosthesis insertion. In addition, the penis can be crushed or lacerated inadvertently by a retractor or sharp instrument, respectively.

Diagnosis

History, Clinical, and Laboratory Findings

- The history and physical examination usually suffice for diagnosing a penile injury.
- With a penile rupture, a popping sound may be reported during intercourse immediately followed by detumescence with ecchymosis and swelling of the penile shaft.
- Injuries from an infectious etiology may present with crepitus, skin necrosis, fever, and leukocytosis. Pathogens responsible for necrotizing infections include *Escherichia coli*, *Bacteroides*, *Streptococcus*, *Klebsiella*, *Staphylococcus*, and *Clostridium*. Common oral pathogens include *Staphylococcus* and *Eikenella corrodens*.

- With penetrating injuries, a laceration or an entrance/exit wound should be readily apparent.
- All other penile injuries are easily identified on inspection (i.e., amputations, constrictions, iatrogenic causes).
- A psychiatric evaluation must be obtained for all self-inflicted penile injuries.

Imaging

- There is a limited role for imaging in the assessment of penile trauma.
- A retrograde urethrogram should be performed for any penile injury, presenting with gross or microscopic hematuria, and in all penetrating injuries.
- Approximately 25 % of penile injuries will have associated urethral injuries.
- Magnetic resonance imaging can be used to confirm a penile rupture when the clinical findings are atypical.

Injury Classification

Penile injuries are classified as follows:

Grade I: cutaneous laceration or contusion

Grade II: laceration of Buck's fascia (cavernosum) without tissue loss

Grade III: cutaneous avulsion, laceration through glans or meatus, or cavernosal or urethral defect <2 cm

Grade IV: partial penectomy or cavernosal or urethral defect = 2 cm

Grade V: total penectomy

Management

Active penile bleeding can usually be controlled with local compression; circumferential compression should be avoided as it will compromise penile blood flow.

The mechanism of injury is important in choosing the appropriate management. Most penile injuries require an operative approach, the goal of which is functional and aesthetic penile restoration. Conservative debridement is advised to preserve as much functional penile tissue as possible.

Ruptures or Fractures
(Zargooshi 2002; Atat et al. 2008) (Fig. 5.37a)

These injuries should be managed with penile exploration and reconstruction to avoid penile curvature from undue scarring.

- The penis should be degloved via a circumferential subcoronal incision, down to Buck's fascia, exposing the entire penile shaft.
- The defect in the tunica albuginea should be identified (Fig. 5.37b) and sutured superficially, avoiding additional injury to the corpus cavernosum.
- A concomitant urethral injury should be recognized and repaired. A partial urethral transection can be approximated with simple sutures, whereas a complete transection requires an anastomotic repair. In both instances, a Foley catheter should be left in place for 1–2 weeks.
- A simulated saline erection can be performed after the repair to ensure penile straightening (Fig. 5.37c).
- A circumcision should be considered, in uncircumcised patients, to avoid significant postoperative foreskin swelling.

Amputations or Mutilations
(Carroll et al. 1985; Jezior et al. 2001)

Successful reimplantation requires the prompt retrieval and proper storage of a salvageable organ and a knowledgeable multidisciplinary reconstructive team.

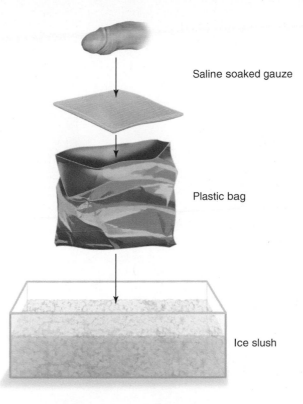

Saline soaked gauze

Plastic bag

Ice slush

FIGURE 5.39 Technique of penile stump storage

- The penile stump should be wrapped in a saline-moistened gauze and placed in a dry container which is then preserved on ice (Fig. 5.39).
- A suprapubic cystotomy should be used for urinary diversion.
- Penile reimplantation is performed by reapproximating the tunica albuginea of the corpora cavernosa (Fig. 5.40a), suturing the urethra (Fig. 5.40b), and microsurgically anastomosing the dorsal artery and vein and nerve, where possible (Fig. 5.40c).

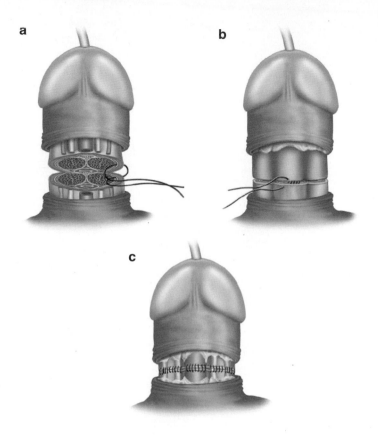

FIGURE 5.40 Penile reimplantation: (**a**) Reapproximation of the corpora cavernosa. (**b**) Urethral anastomosis. (**c**) Microsurgical neurovascular anastomosis

Constrictions

- Constriction ring injuries should be managed with removal of the offending device, local care, and penile elevation. Most will heal without intervention.
- In cases of prolonged penile constriction, interruption of the lymphatic and venous drainage can result in more extensive tissue necrosis complicating recovery. In these cases, penile skin grafting may be required.

Infections

- A suggestion of an infectious etiology mandates aerobic and anaerobic wound cultures and initiation of broad-spectrum antibiotics.
- Tetanus toxoid should be administered for human or animal bites.
- Primary closure of any infected wound is contraindicated.
- Additional principles of management of necrotizing infections include:

  - Immediate fluid and electrolyte resuscitation
  - Repetitive surgical debridement
  - Delayed reconstruction

- Surgical amputation should be avoided. In cases of extensive necrosis, the involved distal penile segment should be allowed to self-amputate.
- Superficial penile burns should be treated with 1 % silver sulfadiazine cream and appropriately covered. Electrical burns usually produce considerable deep tissue damage which may not be readily apparent initially. Nonviable tissue should be debrided cautiously.

Gunshot or Stab Wounds
(Gomez et al. 1993; Kunkle et al. 2008)

Penetrating injuries to the penis should be explored in order to assess the extent of tissue damage. Since most penetrating injuries to the penis occur in polytraumatized patients, it is important to prioritize the injuries by severity. The following techniques are used for penile exploration and reconstruction:

- The penis is explored through a circumcising subcoronal or a penoscrotal incision. Small puncture wounds may be selectively explored locally.
- Minimal debridement is needed in order to avoid further injury to the penis and to facilitate wound closure.
- Closure of the penile and any associated urethral injuries should be completed with absorbable sutures.

Iatrogenic Injuries

Treatment of iatrogenic injuries is dependent on the etiology. Penile reconstructive techniques may be needed to repair extensive skin loss which can occur from overzealous circumcisions and penile augmentation procedures.

Penile Reconstruction

With extensive penile tissue loss, as with burns, necrotizing infections, and overzealous circumcision, various reconstructive techniques can be used depending on the extent of the defect and the experience of the surgeon. It is important to remember that with all infected cases, the initial mainstay of surgical treatment is thorough debridement. All necrotic tissue must be removed, providing a clean host for tissue transplantation.

Total penile skin loss is best managed by split-thickness skin grafting. The graft can be harvested from the anterior lateral thigh at various thicknesses, depending on the local wound conditions and the patient's erectile function. Thinner grafts have improved survival but contract more than thicker grafts and, consequently, may limit subsequent erections. In cases where erectile function is not a concern, the graft can be meshed, facilitating coverage and improving survival.

Full-thickness skin grafts are rarely used in complete penile denudation because of the size of the donor site required and the need for its subsequent closure. For partial penile skin loss, full-thickness skin grafts can be used provided that the donor site is hairless.

Complications

Complications of penile injuries include soft tissue necrosis, erectile dysfunction, penile curvature, loss of penile sensation, urethral stricture, and urethrocutaneous fistula.

Outcome

Penile injuries can be diagnosed easily and should be managed promptly, usually surgically. The details are determined by the mechanism and extent of the injury. The goal of treatment is the preservation of genitourinary function and maintenance of cosmesis. The psychological impact of a poor surgical outcome can be tremendous.

Spinal Cord Injury: Spinal Shock and Autonomic Dysreflexia (Consortium for Spinal Cord Medicine 2001, 2008; Khastgir et al. 2007; Kirshblum et al. 2011)

Spinal cord injury (SCI) usually results from trauma. It is important to know the neurological level and extent of injury. Determining the exact "level" of injury is critical in making accurate predictions about the specific parts of the body that may be affected by paralysis and loss of function, for example, bladder and bowel.

Classification of SCI is based on systematic sensory and motor examination of dermatomes and myotomes to determine the spinal cord segments that are injured. Following the International Standards for Neurological Classification of Spinal Cord Injury (ISNCSCI) guidelines yields the sensory and motor levels of injury (right and left), the neurological level of injury (NLI), sensory scores (pinprick and light touch), motor scores (upper and lower limbs), and the zone of partial preservation (ZPP). The American Spinal Injury Association (ASIA) Impairment Scale (AIS) classifies the severity, or completeness, of injury.

Treatment is based on the advanced trauma life support guidelines including ABCs and resuscitation with initial evaluation and immobilization. There is no clinical evidence to use steroids in this situation. Insert a urethral urinary catheter as part of the initial patient assessment, unless contraindicated. If contraindicated, insert a suprapubic catheter. Leave the indwelling urinary catheter in place at least until the patient is hemodynamically stable. Priapism is usually self-limited in acute SCI and does not require treatment. The body goes into a state of spinal shock within a few minutes of the injury.

Spinal Shock

This is associated with a SCI resulting in a state of sensory and motor loss along with total loss of reflexes following trauma below a specific level due to loss of descending impulses from higher centers. It is important to distinguish this from neurogenic shock which involves hemodynamic instability and is associated with injuries above T6.

In spinal shock, there is an initial increase in blood pressure due to the release of catecholamines, followed by hypotension. Flaccid paralysis, including of the bowel and bladder, is observed, and sometimes sustained priapism develops. Spinal shock is transient, and symptoms tend to last several hours to days until the reflex arcs below the level of the injury begin to function again. It does not indicate circulatory collapse. No specific treatment is required except as above.

There are four phases to spinal shock:

Phase	Time	Physical exam finding	Underlying physiological event
1	0–1 days	Areflexia/hyporeflexia	Loss of descending facilitation
2	1–3 days	Initial reflex return	Denervation supersensitivity
3	1–4 weeks	Hyperreflexia (initial)	Axon-supported synapse growth
4	1–12 months	Hyperreflexia, spasticity	Cell body (soma)-supported synapse growth

Autonomic Dysreflexia

It is a syndrome of massive imbalanced reflex sympathetic discharge, occurring in patients with SCI after the phase of spinal shock in which reflexes return at or above the splanchnic sympathetic outflow (T5–T6). It is more common in cervical (60 %) than thoracic (20 %) injuries. It can occur at any time following the onset of spinal cord paralysis. Patients with incomplete lesions can also experience autonomic dysreflexia but with less severe symptoms.

Pathophysiology of Autonomic Dysreflexia

Below the level of injury, there are intact peripheral sensory nerves transmitting impulses that ascend in the spinothalamic and posterior columns to stimulate sympathetic neurons in the intermediolateral gray matter of the spinal cord. The inhibitory outflow above the SCI from cerebral vasomotor centers is increased, but it is unable to pass below the block of the SCI. Large sympathetic outflow causes release of neurotransmitters (norepinephrine, dopamine) causing piloerection, skin pallor, and severe vasoconstriction in arterial vasculature. This causes a sudden elevation in blood pressure and vasodilation above the level of injury. The vasomotor brainstem reflexes attempt to lower the blood pressure by increasing parasympathetic stimulation to the heart through the vagus nerve to cause compensatory bradycardia but cannot compensate for severe vasoconstriction [Poiseuille law: $\Delta P \propto Q$(bradycardia)$/R^4$ (vasoconstriction)].

The parasympathetic nervous system prevails above the level of injury, causing profuse sweating and vasodilation with skin flushing. The sympathetic nervous system prevails below the level of injury. These result in a sudden rise in both systolic and diastolic blood pressures, usually associated with bradycardia. Normal systolic blood pressure for SCI, above T6, is 90–110 mmHg. A blood pressure of 20–40 mmHg above baseline may be a sign of autonomic dysreflexia.

Signs and Symptoms

Signs

- Flushing and/or blotching and profuse sweating above the level of cord lesion in the face, neck, and shoulders. Rarely below the level of the lesion because of sympathetic cholinergic activity
- Hypertension and bradycardia with pounding, usually frontal, headache (always present)
- Pupillary dilatation, blurred vision, and spots in the visual fields

- Cold peripheries
- Piloerection: goose humps above, or below, level of lesion
- Nasal congestion

Treatment

- Check blood pressure: if elevated and patient is supine, have them sit up immediately and loosen any clothing or constrictive devices. This leads to pooling of the blood into the lower extremities and may reduce blood pressure.
- Monitor blood pressure and pulse rate every 2–5 min until stabilization.
- Use an antihypertensive agent with rapid onset and short duration of action while investigating other causes, for example, give nifedipine 10 mg:

  - Bite and swallow is the preferred method of administration.
  - Beware in the elderly and in patients with coronary artery disease.
  - Treatment may be repeated up to four doses (40 mg) over 1 h.
  - Glyceryl trinitrate (GTN) spray 1–2 doses under the tongue (as alternative to nifedipine).

- Diazepam intravenously for treatment of associated spasms and for control of fits may be useful for control during transfer to a specialist unit.
- Lignocaine gel per rectum/per urethra to block afferent input for 2 min prior to inserting a catheter or doing a rectal examination.
- Pain: do not use aspirin or nonsteroidal anti-inflammatory drugs for analgesia or for relief of headache. Use paracetamol, co-proxamol, and/or consider morphine.
- Remove the cause. Check the urinary system—the most common cause:

  - If there is no indwelling catheter, then catheterize to empty the bladder.

- If there is an indwelling catheter in situ, check for kinks, folds, constrictions, or obstructions and for correct position.
- If the catheter is blocked, gently irrigate the bladder with a small amount of saline/water (10–15 ml) at body temperature. Avoid manually compressing or tapping the bladder.

- If the catheter is draining and the blood pressure remains elevated, suspect fecal impaction (second commonest cause) and do a digital rectal examination using KY jelly or lignocaine gel. If impaction is present, gently carry out a manual evacuation. If the rectum is empty, consider constipation as a cause and arrange appropriate treatment.
- Check the skin for pressure ulcers and abscesses.
- Check for other possible stimuli such as ingrowing toenails, fractures, and deep vein thrombosis and treat accordingly.
- Continue monitoring of symptoms, pulse rate, urinary output, and blood pressure for >2 h after resolution to ensure that elevation of blood pressure does not recur.
- If there is a poor response and/or a cause has not been identified, then refer to medics who may consider:

  - Phentolamine 10 mg/ml ampule, given by intravenous injection, 2–5 mg. This is repeated if necessary. It has a short duration of action. Side effects: tachycardia, dizziness, nausea and vomiting, angina, chest pains, and arrhythmias. Contraindications: hypotension, history of myocardial infarction, and angina.
  - Labetalol 100 mg in 20 ml ampule. Infused at 2 mg/min, until a satisfactory response is obtained. The infusion should then be stopped. Effective dose is usually in the range 50–200 mg. Can be used in pregnancy. Given when the patient is in supine or left lateral position. Raising the patient to an upright position within 3 h of receiving labetalol should be avoided, since excessive postural hypotension may occur. Side effects: excessive hypotension. Contraindications: asthma.
  - Hydralazine: direct acting vasodilator. 20 mg ampule. Given by slow intravenous injection or infusion, 5–10 mg

over 20 min. Repeated if necessary after 20–30 min. Side effects: tachycardia, fluid retention. (Note: alpha blockers may be useful if bladder outlet problems contribute to the dysreflexia.)

• After stabilization, a full review of the patient's care and consideration of precipitating causes should be carried out. This should involve the patient, the family, and all caregivers.
• All patients with a lesion above T6 should be given a written description of autonomic dysreflexia and its treatment and given a personal card to carry at all times.

References

Renal Injuries

Matthews LA, Smith EM, Spirnak JP. Nonoperative treatment of major blunt renal lacerations with urinary extravasation. J Urol. 1997;157:2056–8.

Miller KS, McAninch JW. Radiographic assessment of renal trauma: our 15 year experience. J Urol. 1995;154:352–5.

Morey AF, Bruce JE, McAninch JW. Efficacy of radiographic imaging in pediatric blunt renal trauma. J Urol. 1996;156:2014–8.

Nuss GR, Morey AF, Jenkins AC, Pruitt JH, Dugi III DD, Morse B, Shariat SF. Radiographic predictors of need for angiographic embolization after traumatic renal injury. J Trauma. 2009;67:578–82.

Tillou A, Romero J, Asensio JA, Best CD, Petrone P, Roldon G. Renal vascular injuries. Surg Clin North Am. 2001;81:1417–30.

Toutouzas KG, Karaiskakis M, Kaminski A, Velmahos GC. Nonoperative management of blunt renal trauma: a prospective study. Am Surg. 2002;68:1097–103.

Bleeding Post-Renal Surgery

Baumann C, Westphalen K, Fuchs H, Oesterwitz H, Hierholzer J. Interventional management of renal bleeding after partial nephrectomy. Cardiovasc Intervent Radiol. 2007;30:828–32.

Ginsburg JC, Fransman SL, Singer MA, Cohanim M, Morrin PA. Use of computerized tomography to evaluate bleeding after renal biopsy. Nephron. 1980;26:240–3.

Kessaris DN, Bellman GC, Pardalidis NP, Smith AG. Management of hemorrhage after percutaneous renal surgery. J Urol. 1995;153:604–8.

Richstone L, Reggio E, Ost MC, Seideman C, Fossett LK, Okeke Z, Rastinehad AR, Lobko I, Siegel DN, Smith AD. Hemorrhage following percutaneous renal surgery: characterization of angiographic findings. J Endourol. 2008;22:1129–35.

Acute Renal Artery Occlusion

Blum U, Billmann P, Krause T, Gabelmann A, Keller E, Moser E, Langer M. Effect of local low-dose thrombolysis on clinical outcome in acute embolic renal artery occlusion. Radiology. 1993;189:549–54.

Isles CG, Robertson S, Hill D. Management of renovascular disease: a review of renal artery stenting in 10 studies. QJM. 1999;92:159–67.

Spirnak JP, Resnick MI. Revascularization of traumatic thrombosis of the renal artery. Gynecol Obstet. 1987;164:22–6.

Renal Vein Thrombosis

Laville M, Aguilera D, Maillet PJ, Labeeuw M, Madonna O, Zech P. The prognosis of renal vein thrombosis: a re-evaluation of 27 cases. Nephrol Dial Transplant. 1988;3:247–56.

Llach E, Koffler A, Massry SG. Renal vein thrombosis and the nephritic syndrome. Nephron. 1977;19:65–8.

Zigman A, Yazbeck S, Emil S, Nguyen L. Renal vein thrombosis: a 10-year review. J Pediatr Surg. 2000;35:1540–2.

Ureteral Injuries

Assimos DG, Patterson LC, Taylor CL. Changing incidence and etiology of iatrogenic ureteral injuries. J Urol. 1994;152:2240–6.

Chou MT, Wang CJ, Lien RC. Prophylactic ureteral catheterization in gynecologic surgery: a 12-year randomized trial in a community hospital. Int Urogynecol J. 2009;20:689–93.

Elliot SP, McAninch JW. Ureteral injuries from external violence: a 25 year experience at San Francisco General Hospital. J Urol. 2003;170:1213–6.

Frankman EZ, Wang L, Bunker CH, Lowder JL. Lower urinary tract injury in women in the United States, 1979–2006. AJOG. 2010;495:e1–5.

Ku JH, Kim ME, Jeon YS, Lee NK, Park YH. Minimally invasive management of ureteral injuries recognized late after obstetric and gynecologic surgery. Injury. 2003;34:480–3.

Lask D, Abarbanel J, Luttwak Z, Manes A, Mukamel E. Changing trends in the management of iatrogenic ureteral injuries. J Urol. 1995;154:1693–5.

Perez-Brayfield MR, Keane TE, Krishnan A, Lafontaine P, Feliciano DV, Clarke HS. Gunshot wounds to the ureter: a 40-year experience at Grady Memorial Hospital. J Urol. 2001;166:119–21.

Pelvic Fractures and Injuries to the Urinary System

Demetriades D, Karaiskakis M, Toutouzas K, Alo K, Velmahos G, Chan L. Pelvic fractures: epidemiology and predictors of associated abdominal injuries and outcomes. J Am Coll Surg. 2002;195:1–10.

Koraitim MM, Marzouk ME, Atta MA, Orabi SS. Risk factors and mechanism of urethral injury in pelvic fractures. Br J Urol. 1966;77:876–80.

Ziran BH, Chamberlin E, Shuler FD, Shah M. Delays and difficulties in the diagnosis of lower urologic injuries in the context of pelvic fractures. J Trauma. 2005;58:533–7.

Bladder Injuries

Armenakas NA, Pareek G, Fracchia JA. Iatrogenic bladder perforations: long-term follow-up of 65 patients. J Am Coll Surg. 2004;198:78–82.

Dobrowolski ZF, Lipczynski W, Drewniak T, Jakubik P, Kusionowicz J. External and iatrogenic trauma of the urinary bladder: a survey in Poland. BJU Int. 2002;89:755–6.

Gomez RG, Ceballos L, Coburn M, Corriere JN, Dixon CM, Lobel B, McAninch JW. Consensus statement on bladder injuries. BJU Int. 2004;94:27–32.

Morey AF, Iverson AJ, Swan A, Harmon WJ, Spore SS, Bhayani S, Brandes SB. Bladder rupture after blunt trauma: guidelines for diagnostic imaging. J Trauma. 2001;51:683–6.

Posterior Urethral Injuries

Husmann DA, Wilson WT, Boone TB, Allen TD. Prostatomembranous urethral disruptions: management by suprapubic cystostomy and delayed urethroplasty. J Urol. 1990;144:76–8.

Kizer WS, Armenakas NA, Brandes SB, Cavalcanti AG, Santucci RA, Morey AF. Simplified reconstruction of posterior urethral disruption defects: limited role of supracrural rerouting. J Urol. 2007;177:1378–82.

Mouravier VB, Coburn M, Santucci RA. The treatment of posterior urethral disruption associated with pelvic fractures: comparative experience of early realignment versus delayed urethroplasty. J Urol. 2005;173:873–6.

Perry MO, Husmann DA. Urethral injuries in female subjects following pelvic fractures. J Urol. 1992;147:139–43.

Santucci RA, McAninch JW. Urethral reconstruction of strictures resulting from treatment of benign prostatic hypertrophy and prostate cancer. Urol Clin North Am. 2002;29:417–27.

Venn SN, Greenwell TJ, Mundy AR. Pelvic fracture injuries of the female urethra. BJU Int. 1999;83:626–30.

Webster GD, Ramon J. Repair of pelvic fracture posterior urethral defects using an elaborated perineal approach: experience with 74 cases. J Urol. 1991;145:744–8.

Wessells H, Morey AF, McAninch JW. Obliterative vesicourethral strictures following radical prostatectomy for prostate cancer: reconstructive armamentarium. J Urol. 1998;160:1373–5.

Anterior Urethral Injuries

Husmann DA, Boone TB, Wilson WT. Management of low velocity gunshot wounds of the anterior urethra: the role of primary repair versus urinary diversion alone. J Urol. 1993;150:70–2.

McAninch JW. Traumatic injuries to the urethra. J Trauma. 1981;21:291–7.

Rosenstein DI, Alsikafi NF. Diagnosis and classification of urethral injuries. Urol Clin North Am. 2006;33:73–85.

Testicular Injuries

Buckley JC, McAninch JW. Use of ultrasonography for the diagnosis of testicular injuries in blunt scrotal trauma. J Urol. 2006;175:175–8.

Cass AS. Testicular trauma. J Urol. 1983;129:299–300.

Ferguson GG, Brandes SB. Gunshot wound injury of the testis: the use of tunica vaginalis and polytetrafluoroethylene grafts for reconstruction. J Urol. 2007;178(6):2462–5.

Kudadia AN, Ercole CJ, Gleich P, Hensleigh H, Pryor JL. Testicular trauma: potential impact on reproductive function. J Urol. 1996;156:1643–6.

Phonsombat S, Master VA, McAninch JW. Penetrating external genital trauma: a 30-year single institution experience. J Urol. 2008;180:192–6.

Penile Injuries

Atat RE, Sfaxi M, Benslama MR, Amine D, Ayed M, Mouelli SB, Chebil M, Zmerli S. Fracture of the penis: management and long-term results of surgical treatment. Experience in 300 cases. J Trauma. 2008;64:121–5.

Carroll PR, Lue TF, Schmidt RA, Trengrove-Jones G, McAninch JW. Penile reimplantation: current concepts. J Urol. 1985;133:281–5.

Gomez GR, Castanheira ACC, McAninch JW. J Urol. 1993;150:1147–9.

Jezior JR, Brady J, Schlossberg SM. Management of penile amputation injuries. World J Surg. 2001;25:1602–9.

Kunkle DA, Lehed BD, Mydlo JH, Pontari MA. Evaluation and management of gunshot wounds of the penis: 20 year experience at an urban trauma center. J Trauma. 2008;64:1038–42.

Zargooshi J. Penile fracture in Kermanshah, Iran: the long-term results of surgical treatment. BJU Int. 2002;89:890–4.

Spinal Cord Injury: Spinal Shock and Autonomic Dysreflexia

Consortium for Spinal Cord Medicine. Acute management of autonomic dysreflexia: individuals with spinal cord injury presenting to health-care facilities. 2nd ed. Washington, DC: Consortium for Spinal Cord Medicine Clinical Practice Guidelines; 2001.

Consortium for Spinal Cord Medicine. Early acute management in adults with spinal cord injury: a clinical practice guideline for health-care professionals. J Spinal Cord Med. 2008;31(4):403–79.

http://www.spinalunit.scot.nhs.uk/Spinal%20Documents/AUTDYS.pdf

Khastgir J, Drake MJ, Abrams P. Recognition and effective management of autonomic dysreflexia in spinal cord injuries. Expert Opin Pharmacother. 2007;8(7):945–56.

Kirshblum SC, Burns SP, Biering-Sorensen F, et al. International standards for neurological classification of spinal cord injury (revised 2011). J Spinal Cord Med. 2011;34(6):535–46.

Chapter 6
Scrotal and Genital Emergencies

John Reynard

Torsion of the Testis and Testicular Appendages

During fetal development, the testis descends into the inguinal canal and as it does so it pushes in front of it a covering of peritoneum (Fig. 6.1). This covering of peritoneum, which actually forms a tube, is called the processus vaginalis. The testis lies behind this tube of peritoneum, and by birth, or shortly afterward, the lumen of the tube becomes obliterated. In the scrotum, the tube of peritoneum is called the tunica vaginalis. The testis essentially is pushed into the tunica vaginalis from behind. The tunica vaginalis, therefore, is actually two layers of peritoneum, which cover the testis everywhere apart from its most posterior surface (Fig. 6.2). The layer of peritoneum that is in direct contact with the testis is called the visceral layer of the tunica vaginalis, and the layer that surrounds this and actually covers the inner surface of the scrotum is called the parietal layer of the tunica vaginalis.

J. Reynard, DM, FRCS (Urol)
Department of Urology, Nuffield Department of Surgical Sciences,
Oxford University Hospitals, Oxford, UK

The National Spinal Injuries Centre, Stoke Mandeville Hospital,
Aylesbury, UK
e-mail: john.reynard@ouh.nhs.uk

H. Hashim et al. (eds.), *Urological Emergencies* 181
In Clinical Practice, DOI 10.1007/978-1-4471-2720-8_6,
© Springer-Verlag London 2013

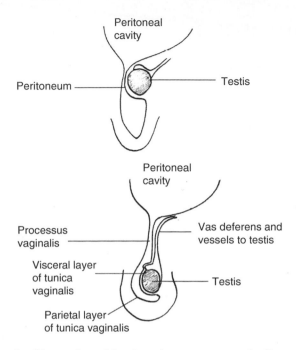

FIGURE 6.1 The testis pushing into the processus vaginalis

In the neonate, the parietal layer of the tunica vagina-lis may not have firmly fused with the other layers of the scrotum, and therefore, it is possible for the tunica vaginalis and the contained testis to twist within the scrotum. This is called an extravaginal torsion, i.e., the twist occurs *outside* of the two layers of the tunica vaginalis. In boys and men, the parietal layer of the tunica vaginalis has fused with the other layers of the scrotum. Thus, an extravaginal torsion cannot occur.

In most boys and men, the testis is covered on its front and sides by the visceral layer of the tunica vaginalis, but its pos-terior surface is not so covered, and the posterior surface of the testis is therefore in direct contact with, and fused to, the layers of the posterior scrotum. Being fused to the scrotum in

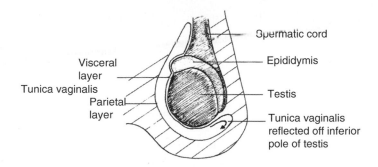

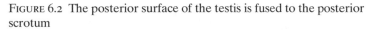

FIGURE 6.2 The posterior surface of the testis is fused to the posterior scrotum

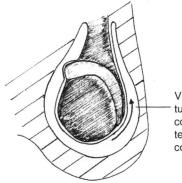

Visceral layer of tunica vaginalis covering the entire testis and spermatic cord

FIGURE 6.3 The entire surface of the testis together with a length of the spermatic cord is covered with the visceral layer of the tunica vaginalis. This is the bell clapper, and it predisposes to intravaginal torsion of the testis and epididymis

this way, the testis cannot twist around (Fig. 6.2). However, in some boys and men, the entire surface of the testis, together with a length of the spermatic cord, is covered with the visceral layer the tunica vaginalis (Fig. 6.3). In these individuals, the testis hangs like the clapper of a bell within the scrotum. It is therefore free to rotate within the scrotum. This is called an intravaginal torsion, i.e., it occurs *between* the two layers of the tunica vaginalis.

Testicular Appendages

Attached to the testis are so-called testicular appendages. These are vestigial and are derived from embryological structures. The appendix testis (also known as a hydatid of Morgagni) is a remnant of the Müllerian duct (in the female fetus this develops into the fallopian tubes and upper part of the vagina). In 80 % of individuals, it is pedunculated (Rolnick et al. 1968) (i.e., it is on a stalk) and is therefore prone to torsion, which can cause pain (mimicking that of a testicular torsion).

The epididymis, vas deferens, and seminal vesicles are derived from the mesonephric (Wolffian) duct. An appendix epididymis, not surprisingly, is a derivative of the Wolffian duct (more specifically a remnant of a cranial mesonephric tubule) and it is almost always pedunculated. Like an appendix testis, the appendix epididymis may twist and cause scrotal pain.

Definition

A testicular torsion is a twist of the spermatic cord resulting in strangulation of the blood supply to the testis and epididymis. It is a vascular emergency! It may be (a) intravaginal where the testis twists within the tunica vaginalis, the more common type, or (b) extravaginal, the type that occurs in the neonatal or prenatal period.

Testicular torsion occurs most frequently between the ages of 10 and 30, with a peak at the age of 13–15 years, but any age group may be affected. The left side is said to be affected more often, and 2 % are said to present with torsion of both testes.

Presentation

The presentation is usually one of sudden onset of severe pain in the hemiscrotum, sometimes waking the patient from sleep. It may radiate to the groin or loin, reflecting the embryological origin of the testis and its nerve supply. In some patients the loin, groin, or abdominal pain may so dominate that the patient may fail to mention (or may not even notice) that they have scrotal pain, and the unwary doctor may therefore fail to examine the scrotum.

Nausea and vomiting are common.

There may be a history of a blow to the testis in the hours before the acute onset of pain. Some patients report similar episodes occurring in the past, with spontaneous resolution of the pain, suggesting an episode of torsion with spontaneous detorsion. The patient will be in considerable pain and may have a slight fever. Patients do not like the testis being touched and will find it difficult to walk and to get up on the examination couch, as movement causes pain. The testis is usually swollen, very tender to touch, and may appear abnormally tense (if the patient lets you squeeze it!). It may be high-riding (lying at a higher than normal position in the testis) and may be in a horizontal position due to twisting of the cord. The testis may feel hard and there may be scrotal wall erythema.

The cremasteric reflex may be lost, although the presence or absence of this reflex should not be taken as reliable evidence either that the patient has a torsion or does not (Nelson et al. 2003). The cremasteric reflex may be elicited by stroking the finger along the inside of the thigh, which results in upward movement of the ipsilateral testis.

Differential Diagnosis

This includes epididymo-orchitis and torsion of a testicular appendage and causes of flank pain with radiation into the groin and testis. From time to time, the pain of a ureteric stone may be localized to the ipsilateral testis, but when the testis is palpated, the patient has no tenderness. In such cases a plain computed tomography (CT-KUB) confirms the presence of a stone.

Clinically, the pain of a twisted appendix testis or appendix epididymis can be difficult to distinguish from that of a testicular torsion. Sometimes, though, a little boy presents with scrotal pain and the area of tenderness on examination of the

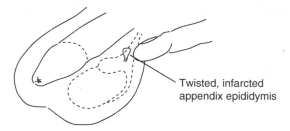

Twisted, infarcted
appendix epididymis

FIGURE 6.4 Point tenderness in a case of a twisted appendix epididymis

scrotum is confined almost to a single spot, which can be localized by the tip of the examining finger (Fig. 6.4). We have never felt comfortable relying on this sign to exclude a testicular torsion and have always explored such cases.

Investigations

Both color Doppler ultrasound and radionuclide scanning can be used to diagnose testicular torsion (Al Mufti et al. 1995; Melloul et al. 1995). Color Doppler ultrasound shows reduced arterial blood flow in the testicular artery. While intra-testicular blood flow is absent in most affected torted testes, a significant minority have persistent arterial inflow. In Kalfa's study (Kalfa et al. 2004), 31 of 44 cases had absent flow, but flow was present in 13 of 44 cases – so color Doppler ultrasound scanning "missed" the diagnosis in 13 (30 %) of 44 cases.

Surgical Management

The mainstay of investigation and treatment of a suspected case of testicular torsion remains, in many hospitals, scrotal exploration. This should be undertaken as a matter of urgency. Delay in relieving the twisted testis can result in permanent ischemic damage to the testis with subsequent atrophy, loss of hormone production, and loss of sperm production. Furthermore, as the testis undergoes necrosis, the blood–testis barrier breaks down and an autoimmune reaction has been shown to develop (sympathetic orchidopathia) in animal models (Cerasaro et al. 1984; Wallace et al. 1982). Whether this occurs in humans to the extent that spermatogenesis is impaired is uncertain (Anderson and Williamson 1986). The autoantibodies so produced can then damage the contralateral testis, thereby impairing hormone production and spermatogenesis of this side as well. A delay in relieving the torsion of more than 6 h increases the risk that ischemic necrosis will take place.

In a series of 670 patients with testicular torsion from Bristol in the UK, Anderson and Williamson (1988) demonstrated that if surgery was performed within 6 h, only 2 % of testes were nonviable at operation. If surgery was performed between 7 and 12 h following the onset of symptoms, 90 % of testicles were "saved" and 10 % were nonviable.

Watkin and colleagues (1996) from Bath reported outcomes of surgical treatment of testicular torsion in a series of 71 patients (see Table 6.1).

This study demonstrated that where exploration of the testicle was delayed for between 8 and 16 h after onset of testicular pain, the testicular salvage rate fell from 100 % (for those operated on within 4 h) to 75 %.

Warn the patient (and if he is a child, warn his parents) that if the testis is found to be dead at exploration, the best thing to do is to remove it. This is done to reduce the likelihood of an autoimmune reaction affecting the normal contralateral testis but also because this provides the best pain relief and prevents the potential complication of infection of the necrotic tissue (which could lead to subsequent abscess formation).

Under general anesthesia, the scrotum is explored. We use a midline incision, since this allows access to both sides so that they may both be "fixed" within the scrotum. In some cases, the testis may already be black and obviously necrotic. The spermatic cord should be ligated with a transfixion stitch of an absorbable material, and the testis should be removed. If the testis has twisted and appears

TABLE 6.1 Percentage salvage rate of testicles operated on for testicular torsion, according to symptom duration (defined as time of onset of testicular symptoms) versus onset of anesthetic for surgical exploration

Symptom duration (h)	Number of viable testes	Orchidectomy	Percentage of testicles operated on as a % of total	Testis salvage rate (%)
0–4	12	0	17	100
4.1–8	28	3	44	90
8.1–16	9	3	17	75
>16	4	12	22	25
Overall salvage rate				75

Modified from Watkin et al. (1996)

to be viable, untwist it and wait for it to "pink up." Give it the benefit of the doubt. Wait 10 min, placing the testis in a warm swab. You can use this timing to fix the other side. If, after 10 min, the viability of the testis is in doubt, make a small cut with the tip of a scalpel. If the testis bleeds actively, it should be salvaged (close the small wound with an absorbable suture).

There is some controversy surrounding the best technique for fixation. Some surgeons fix the testis within the scrotum with suture material, inserted at two or three points. Those who recommend three-point fixation do so because they argue it reduces the risk of retorsion (Phipps 1987; Thurston and Whitaker 1983). Some use absorbable sutures and others nonabsorbable sutures. Those who use the latter argue that absorbable sutures may disappear, exposing the patient to the risk of subsequent retorsion. Indeed, in a literature review, Kuntze et al. (1985) found that 15 of 16 patients with recurrent torsion had undergone previous orchidopexy using absorbable suture material, and they recommended the use of 2/0 or 3/0 nonabsorbable suture material. Those who use absorbable sutures argue that the fibrous reaction around the absorbable sutures used to fix the testis will prevent retorsion and that the patient may be able to feel nonabsorbable sutures, which can be uncomfortable (though this should not occur if the sutures are placed medially, i.e., into the septum between the two testes). If you use suture fixation, these should pass through the visceral layer of the tunica vaginalis covering the testis, through the tough tunica albuginea of the testis, and then through the parietal layer of the tunica vaginalis, which lines the inner surface of the scrotum. We find it easier to clip each suture and to tie them only after all three have been placed. Tying them after each has been placed can make it difficult to insert the next suture.

Other surgeons have argued that the testis should be fixed within a dartos pouch (Frank and O'Brien 2002). The rationale behind this form of fixation is that suture fixation breaches the blood–testis barrier, thereby exposing both testes to the risk of sympathetic orchidopathia. Dartos pouch fixation should, in theory, avoid this potential risk. In a review of 387 patients who had undergone unilateral or bilateral orchidopexy, Coughlin et al. (1998) reported that the use of testicular suture material was strongly associated with infertility. Concerns have also been expressed about a possible increased cancer risk in testes that have been suture fixed (Frank and O'Brien 2002).

Many surgeons continue to use suture fixation, and indeed operative surgery textbooks still describe this technique for use in testicular fixation for torsion (Hinman 1998).

If you use dartos pouch fixation, open the tunica vaginalis, bring the testis out, and untwist it. Develop a dartos pouch in the scrotum by holding the skin with forceps and dissecting with scissors between the skin and the underlying dartos muscle. Once you have started to develop this space, it can be enlarged by inserting your two index fingers and pulling them apart. Place the testis in this pouch. A few absorbable sutures may be used to attach the cord near the testis to the inside of the dartos pouch. This can help to prevent retorsion of the testes (which we have seen in testes that have been placed in a dartos pouch). The dartos may then be closed over the testis and the skin can be closed in a separate layer.

Whatever technique you use, remember to fix *both* testes since the bell-clapper abnormality, which predisposes to torsion, can occur bilaterally.

If we find an appendix testis or appendix epididymis at the time of scrotal exploration, whether there is a testicular torsion or not, we remove it (with diathermy or by ligating it with a small suture), so that it cannot twist in the future, which would necessitate repeat scrotal exploration.

If we find that the testis is not twisted, then we assume that the testis had undergone torsion, but had untwisted once the patient had been anesthetized, or that the diagnosis could be epididymo-orchitis. If there was free fluid surrounding the testis, we take a swab and send it for culture. We fix the testis and the contralateral testis as a prophylactic measure.

Priapism

Definition

Persistent erection of the penis (full or partial) for more than 4 h that is not related or accompanied by sexual desire. There are two main types: *ischemic* (veno-occlusive, low flow) and *nonischemic* (arterial, high flow – essentially trauma related). It can affect any age, but the two main age groups affected are 5- to 10-year-old boys and 20- to 50-year-old men. There is a third type of priapism called *stuttering priapism*, which is an intermittent recurrent form of ischemic priapism, historically described in the context of recurrent, painful, and unwanted erections in the context of sickle cell disease.

History

Questions you should ask:

Duration of erection >4 h?
Is it painful or not? Pain implies ischemia due to low flow; absence of pain implies high-flow priapism with no ischemia (often onset of priapism delayed by many hours after trauma). Any history of perineal or penile trauma?
Previous history and treatment of priapism?

Direct your questions toward predisposing conditions and factors:

- Drugs: Alpha-blockers; antidepressants and antipsychotics; antihypertensives – propranolol, hydralazine, and guanethidine; recreational drugs – cocaine and marijuana; testosterone therapy; vasoactive erectile drugs – papaverine, phentolamine, prostaglandin E1, oral phosphodiesterase inhibitors (rare, though more likely in men with other predisposing conditions, e.g., spinal injury, sickle cell disease, and those on antipsychotic drugs)
- Trauma: straddle injury, coital injury, pelvic trauma, and blow to perineum or penis (leading to laceration of cavernosal

artery within the corpora or a branch of a cavernosal artery; this causes uncontrolled pooling of blood in sinusoidal spaces – a cavernosal-sinusoidal fistula)

- Iatrogenic trauma: optical urethrotomy, Nesbit's corporoplasty, and postsurgical shunting or even post-alpha-adrenergic injection for low-flow priapism (i.e., conversion of low- to high-flow priapism)
- Neurological: cerebrovascular accident, lumbar disc prolapse, and spinal cord injury
- Hematologic disease: sickle cell; thalassemia; leukemia; myeloma
- Neoplastic: (metastatic or local infiltration) prostate, urethra, testis, bladder, rectum, lung, and kidney

Examination

Look for the following:

Rigid corpora cavernosa
The corpus spongiosum and glans penis are usually flaccid
Tender penis implies ischemic priapism; non-tender nonischemic priapism

Rarely – perineal or penile bruising indicating trauma; malignant nodules infiltrating the corporal bodies

Investigations

- Full blood count (white blood cell count and differential, reticulocyte count).
- Hemoglobin electrophoresis for sickle cell test.
- Urinalysis including urine toxicology.
- Blood gases taken from either corpora, using a blood gas syringe to aspirate blood, will help in differentiating between low-flow (dark blood; $pH < 7.25$ (acidosis); $pO_2 < 30$ mmHg (hypoxia); $pCO_2 > 60$ mmHg (hypercapnia)) and high-flow priapism (bright red blood similar to arterial blood at room temperature; $pH = 7.4$; $pO_2 > 90$ mmHg; $pCO_2 < 40$ mmHg).

- Color flow duplex ultrasonography in cavernosal arteries: ischemic (inflow low or nonexistent) versus nonischemic (inflow normal to high). This investigation may not be available at all hours.
- Penile pudendal arteriography may be done but is not readily available at all hours.

Treatment

Treatment depends on the type of priapism. Conservative treatment should be tried first, and if it fails, then it is followed by medical treatment (oral sympathomimetics, e.g., terbutaline, pseudoephrine) if the priapism has been of short (<4 h) duration or minimally invasive treatment (aspiration +/– intracavernosal sympathomimetics) and then by surgical treatment (Table 6.2).

Aspiration

Place the butterfly needle into one or other corpora at the penoscrotal junction in 3-o'clock or 9-o'clock positions to avoid the dorsal neurovascular bundles.

Aspirate dark red (deoxygenated blood) until oxygenated (bright red) blood is seen.

Note: It is important to warn all patients with priapism of the possibility of impotence. It should be recorded in the notes and clearly written on the discharge instruction sheet.

Surgical Management of Ischemic Priapism

Indicated where repeated aspiration and injection of sympathomimetic drugs have failed to resolve the ischemic priapism (Keoghane et al. 2002).

It involves creation of a fistula between the corpora cavernosa and (a) the corpus spongiosum or (b) the saphenous vein by a variety of eponymous procedures. For the percutaneous techniques, use a penile ring block or a spinal or general anesthetic.

TABLE 6.2 Treatment algorithm for priapism

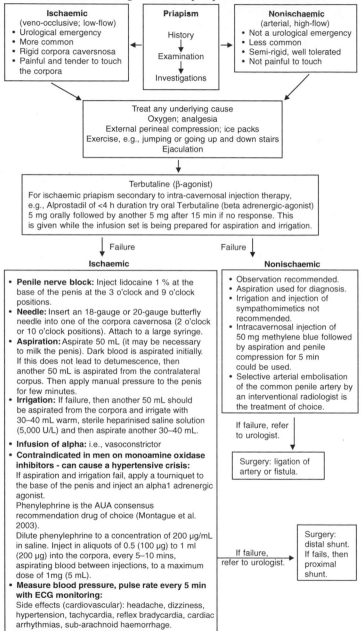

Percutaneous Corporoglanular (Cavernoglanular) Shunt

Winter: transglanular insertion of a large bore needle or Venflon

Ebbehoj: transglanular insertion of a no.11 scalpel blade so developing a straight incision between the glans (corpus spongiosum) and corpus cavernosum. Milk deoxygenated blood out of the open wound until bright red oxygenated blood is obtained. Perform bilateral incisions if required to achieve detumescence. Close the skin with 4/0 Vicryl.

T-shunt: transglanular insertion of a no.10 scalpel blade from the glans (corpus spongiosum) into the corpus cavernosum, which is then rotated 90° and withdrawn. Milk deoxygenated blood out of the open wound until bright red oxygenated blood is obtained. Perform bilateral incisions if required to achieve detumescence. Close the skin with 4/0 Vicryl.

Open Corporoglanular Shunt (Cavernoglanular) (Al-Ghorab)

Excision of a segment of the tunica of the corpus spongiosum in the glans thereby creating a shunt between the corpus spongiosum and the corpus cavernosum.

Open Proximal Shunt

Creation of a shunt between the corpus spongiosum and corpus cavernosum (Quackels) (bilateral "staggered" shunts, i.e., not at the same level – to reduce urethral stricture risk – may be required). It is done via a perineal or transcrotal approach.

Saphenous Vein Shunt (Grayhack)

Anastomosis of the saphenous vein to the corporus cavernosum.

Paraphimosis

Definition

This is a condition in which the foreskin is retracted from over the glans of the penis and cannot then be pulled back over the glans into its normal anatomical position. Essentially the foreskin becomes trapped behind the glans of the penis. It can affect males at any age, but it occurs most commonly in teenagers or young men. It also occurs in elderly men who have had the foreskin retracted during catheterization but not been returned to its normal position after catheterization. It can occur in an otherwise normal foreskin, which if left in the retracted position may become edematous to the point where it cannot be reduced. Occasionally a phimotic foreskin (a tight foreskin that is difficult to retract off the glans) is retracted, and it is then impossible for it to be put back in its normal position.

History

Ask the patient if he is normally able to retract the foreskin (suggesting an otherwise normal foreskin if he can and a phimotic one if he cannot).

Examination

Paraphimosis is usually painful. The foreskin is edematous. It may become so engorged with edema fluid that the appearance can be very confusing for those who have never seen it. Occasionally in a paraphimosis that has been present for several days, a small area of ulceration of the foreskin may have developed, which those unfamiliar with the condition may misinterpret as a malignant or infective process.

Treatment

There are several options. The patient will probably already have tried the application of pressure to the edematous foreskin in an attempt to reduce it, and usually the attending doctor does the same, sometimes successfully reducing the foreskin, but more often than not failing to do so.

The "iced-glove" method (Houghton 1973): Apply topical lignocaine (lidocaine) gel to the glans and foreskin. Wait for 5 min so you achieve anesthesia of the area. Place ice and water in a rubber glove and tie a knot in the cuff of the glove to prevent the contents from pouring out. Also tie off the four fingers of the glove. Place the thumb of the glove over the penis so that the penis lies within it and in contact with the ice and water. This may reduce the swelling and allow reduction of the foreskin.

Granulated sugar has been used to reduce the edema (by an osmotic effect). The sugar may be placed in a condom or glove applied over the end of the penis. The process of reduction may take several hours (Kerwat et al. 1998).

Hyaluronidase injections have been used (1 mL; 150 U/cc), injected via a 25-gauge hypodermic needle into the prepuce. This breaks down hyaluronic acid and decreases the edema (De Vries et al. 1996).

The Dundee technique (Reynard and Barua 1999): Give the patient a broad-spectrum antibiotic such as 500 mg of ciprofloxacin by mouth. Apply a ring block to the base of the penis using a 26-gauge needle. Use 10 mL of 1 % plain lidocaine or 10–20 mL of 0.5 % plain bupivacaine (Marcaine) to the skin at the base of the penis. Wait for 5 min. Touch the skin of the prepuce to check that the penis has been anesthetized. Try pricking the skin of the penis with a sterile needle and ask the patient if he can feel it to make sure it is well anesthetized. Occasionally adequate anesthesia is not achieved and the patient will require a general anesthetic. In children we have tended to use general anesthesia. Clean the skin of the foreskin and the glans with cleaning solution. Using a 25-gauge needle, make approximately 20 punctures into the edematous foreskin. Firmly squeeze the foreskin. This forces the edema fluid out of the foreskin (Fig. 6.5). Small "jets" of edema fluid will be seen. Once the foreskin has been decompressed, it can usually be returned to its normal position. We discharge the patient on a 7-day course of ciprofloxacin as a prophylactic measure and recommend daily baths with careful cleaning of the glans and skin with soap and water. The patient should be advised to dry the foreskin carefully and return it to its normal position afterward.

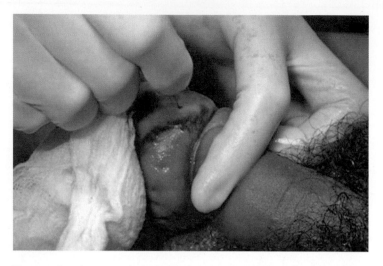

FIGURE 6.5 A case of paraphimosis undergoing reduction by the Dundee technique

Since we first used the Dundee technique in 1996, we have not had to perform a dorsal slit in any patient (Reynard and Barua 1999). We have used this method of reduction in cases where the paraphimosis had been present for a week. Approximately one third of patients underwent elective circumcision for an underlying phimosis.

If this method fails to reduce the paraphimosis, then recourse to the traditional surgical treatment of a dorsal slit is required, usually under general anesthetic or ring block. Make an incision in the tight band of constricting tissue. Pull the foreskin back over the glans, checking that it can move easily over the glans. If you make a longitudinal incision, this may be closed transversely, so essentially lengthening the circumference of the foreskin and hopefully preventing further recurrences of the paraphimosis (Fig. 6.6).

If, having had a dorsal slit, the patient is concerned about the cosmetic appearance or if the underlying cause of the paraphimosis was a phimosis, then he may undergo circumcision at a later date. We have avoided immediate circumcision in such cases because the gross distortion of the normal

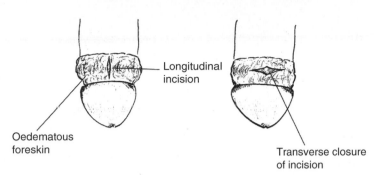

Longitudinal incision

Oedematous foreskin

Transverse closure of incision

FIGURE 6.6 A dorsal slit with the longitudinal incision closed transversely

anatomy of the foreskin can make circumcision difficult and lead to a less than perfect cosmetic result.

Foreign Bodies in the Urethra and Attached to the Penis

All manner of foreign bodies have been inserted into the urethra and bladder either voluntarily, by accident, or as a consequence of assault (van Ophoven and de Kernion 2000; Osca et al. 1991). Most "find" their way into the urethra or bladder in the search for sexual gratification. Occasionally elderly patients with dementia insert objects into their urethra and from time to time catheters and endoscopic equipment (e.g., the insulated tip of a resectoscope) may be "lost" within the urethra or bladder.

History

Patients may present either acutely or months or even years after the object was inserted. They may complain of pain on voiding or suprapubic pain; they may report episodes of hematuria or may present in urinary retention. The patient may volunteer that they have inserted something into the urethra, but sometimes no such history is forthcoming.

Examination and Investigations

The object may be protruding from the ureth
you may be able to feel it within the urethra. A
the pelvis and genitalia may locate the foreign
radiopaque. Alternatively, an ultrasound can loc
If no foreign body is seen ascending, urethrogra
cystoscopy can be used to identify its presence

Treatment

Removing the foreign body can be a challenge
1999). Occasionally it may be voided spontaneo
often than not you have to go in after it. Atte
made to remove it using a flexible cystoscope
and small enough to be grasped in a stone bask
with forceps, but the latter usually cannot appl
chase on the object to allow it to be drawn all
of urethra. It may be possible to retrieve the obj
eral anesthetic using a rigid cystoscope or wider
scope. If this fails, then open cystostomy will be
object is made of glass, such as a thermometer,
safer to avoid the attempt to remove it per the u
of the danger that it might break and damage
even become lodged within the urethra. A form
tomy may be safer for retrieval of glass objects.

If the foreign body is lying within the urethr
be pulled out or pushed back into the bladder (
by rigid cystoscopy or open cystostomy), a ure
have to be performed in order to extract it.

Foreign bodies that have been attached to
as rings, may be particularly difficult to remo
they are made of steel. The object may have be
from view by penile swelling, in which case th
sues will have to be divided to allow the obje
A technique for removing rings from fin
adopted for those stuck on the penis. A silk s

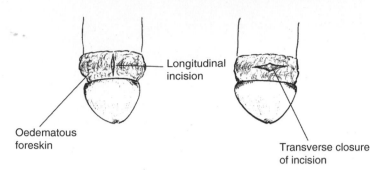

Longitudinal incision

Oedematous foreskin

Transverse closure of incision

FIGURE 6.6 A dorsal slit with the longitudinal incision closed transversely

anatomy of the foreskin can make circumcision difficult and lead to a less than perfect cosmetic result.

Foreign Bodies in the Urethra and Attached to the Penis

All manner of foreign bodies have been inserted into the urethra and bladder either voluntarily, by accident, or as a consequence of assault (van Ophoven and de Kernion 2000; Osca et al. 1991). Most "find" their way into the urethra or bladder in the search for sexual gratification. Occasionally elderly patients with dementia insert objects into their urethra and from time to time catheters and endoscopic equipment (e.g., the insulated tip of a resectoscope) may be "lost" within the urethra or bladder.

History

Patients may present either acutely or months or even years after the object was inserted. They may complain of pain on voiding or suprapubic pain; they may report episodes of hematuria or may present in urinary retention. The patient may volunteer that they have inserted something into the urethra, but sometimes no such history is forthcoming.

Examination and Investigations

The object may be protruding from the urethral meatus or you may be able to feel it within the urethra. A plain X-ray of the pelvis and genitalia may locate the foreign body if it is radiopaque. Alternatively, an ultrasound can locate the object. If no foreign body is seen ascending, urethrography or flexible cystoscopy can be used to identify its presence and location.

Treatment

Removing the foreign body can be a challenge (Johnin et al. 1999). Occasionally it may be voided spontaneously, but more often than not you have to go in after it. Attempts may be made to remove it using a flexible cystoscope if it is smooth and small enough to be grasped in a stone basket or grabbed with forceps, but the latter usually cannot apply enough purchase on the object to allow it to be drawn all of the way out of urethra. It may be possible to retrieve the object under general anesthetic using a rigid cystoscope or wider-bore resectoscope. If this fails, then open cystostomy will be required. If the object is made of glass, such as a thermometer, then it may be safer to avoid the attempt to remove it per the urethra because of the danger that it might break and damage the urethra or even become lodged within the urethra. A formal open cystostomy may be safer for retrieval of glass objects.

If the foreign body is lying within the urethra and it cannot be pulled out or pushed back into the bladder (to be retrieved by rigid cystoscopy or open cystostomy), a urethrostomy will have to be performed in order to extract it.

Foreign bodies that have been attached to the penis, such as rings, may be particularly difficult to remove, especially if they are made of steel. The object may have become obscured from view by penile swelling, in which case the overlying tissues will have to be divided to allow the object to be seen. A technique for removing rings from fingers has been adopted for those stuck on the penis. A silk suture is passed underneath the ring, and the remainder of the suture is then bound tightly around the glans. The proximal end of the suture is then lifted and unwound from the penis, and as this is done the encircling object may be gently pushed distally over the glans, which has been wrapped in the suture.

Alternatively, files, oscillating saws (used to remove plaster casts), or strong bone-cutting forceps may be required to remove the object – call a friendly orthopedic surgical colleague who no doubt will be delighted to assist you! If it is made of steel, a high-speed drill, such as a dentist's drill, may be needed to cut it off. These drills can generate a substantial amount of heat as they cut through the metal, and the penis will need to be cooled with saline irrigation as the procedure is carried out and protected by the use of tongue depressors, for example. Occasionally the equipment and help of the fire brigade may need to be called upon to cut through steel rings when standard hospital drills are not man enough for the job.

Vesicovaginal Fistula: Acute Management

In the Western world, vesicovaginal fistula occurs following hysterectomy, the mechanism being (a) an unrecognized bladder injury, following which urine leaks through the hole in the bladder and exits through the suture line of the vaginal closure; (b) a recognized bladder injury which is repaired at the time, but where the repair then subsequently breaks down; (c) placement of sutures between the vaginal cuff and back wall of the bladder during vaginal closure at the time of hysterectomy. Tissue necrosis then occurs around the sutures leading to development of a fistula between the bladder and the vagina; and (d) a diathermy burn to the bladder occurring at the time of the hysterectomy, which then subsequently undergoes necrosis.

The patient presents with a vaginal leak of urine. Cystoscopy may demonstrate an obvious, usually midline fistula. Instillation of methylene blue through the cystoscope (or a catheter) will exit through the fistula and will stain a pad placed high within the vagina.

"Emergency" management in the form of catheter insertion is usually a temporizing measure prior to definitive surgical repair. However, if inserted less than 3 weeks following the initial injury, as many as 39 % (22 of 57) of women experience spontaneous VVF closure – so a significant minority of patients may experience spontaneous closure, but most did not (Bazi 2007). When a catheter is inserted more than 6 weeks after the insult, only 1 (3 %) of 32 VVF spontaneously healed.

Early (within 3 weeks) catheter drainage may thus lead to spontaneous healing of a fistula where this is small and the patient is continent after placement of an indwelling catheter.

Infection of Prosthetics: The Artificial Urinary Sphincter and Penile Implants

Infections of both devices share common themes. Both can become infected early (within the first few weeks postimplantation) or late (between 6 months and 2 years). The former are derived from bacterial contamination at the time of surgery and are usually gram-negative organisms (Kabalin and Kessler 1988; Licht et al. 1995). The latter are usually gram-positive organisms (*Staph. epidermidis*, *Staph. aureus*) and may be blood borne (Carson and Robertson 1988). Diabetes may increase the risk of infection. Implants in spinal cord injury patients are definitely at greater risk of infection.

Symptoms and signs include scrotal and/or perineal pain, fever, erythema, and tenderness of the skin over the infected component, e.g., the pump located within the scrotum, discharge of pus from the incision site or from the skin overlying the pump, and erosion of the pump through the scrotal skin.

Antibiotics alone are rarely enough to treat the infection, removal of all the components of the penile prosthesis or artificial sphincter almost always being required since bacteria are shielded from antibiotics by a biofilm.

References

Al Mufti RA, Ogedegbe AK, Lafferty K. The use of Doppler ultrasound in the clinical management of acute testicular pain. Br J Urol. 1995;76:625–7.

Anderson JB, Williamson RCN. The fate of the human testis following unilateral torsion of the spermatic cord. Br J Urol. 1986;58:698–704.

Anderson JB, Williamson RCN. Testicular torsion in Bristol: a 25 year review. Br J Surg. 1988;75:988–92.

Bazi T. Spontaneous closure of vesicovaginal fistulas after bladder drainage alone: review of the evidence. Int Urogynecol J Pelvic Floor Dysfunct. 2007;18:329–33.

Carson CC, Robertson CN. Late hematogenous infection of penile prostheses. J Urol. 1988;139:50–2.

Cerasaro TG, Nachtscheim DA, Otero F, Parsons L. The effect of testicular torsion on contralateral testis and the production of antisperm antibodies in rabbits. J Urol. 1984;135:577–9.

Coughlin HT, Bellinger MF, La Porte RE, Lee PA. Testicular suture: a significant risk factor for infertility among formerly cryptorchid men. J Pediatr Surg. 1998;33:1790–3.

De Vries CR, Miller AK, Packer MG. Reduction of paraphimosis with hyaluronidase. Urology. 1996;48:464–5.

Frank JD, O'Brien M. Related articles, fixation of the testis. Br J Urol Int. 2002;89:331–3.

Hinman Jr F. Atlas of urologic surgery. Philadelphia: WB Saunders; 1998.

Houghton GR. The 'iced-glove' method of treatment of paraphimosis. Br J Surg. 1973;60:876–7.

Johnin K, Kushima M, Koizumi S, et al. Percutaneous transvesical retrieval of foreign bodies penetrating the urethra. J Urol. 1999;161:915–6.

Kabalin JN, Kessler R. Infectious complications of penile prosthesis surgery. J Urol. 1988;139:953–5.

Kalfa N, Veyrac C, Baud C, Couture A, Averous M, Galifer RB. Ultrasonography of the spermatic cord in children with testicular torsion: impact on the surgical strategy. J Urol. 2004;172:1692–5.

Keoghane SR, Sullivan ME, Miller MA. The aetiology, pathogenesis and management of priapism. Br J Urol Int. 2002;90:149–54.

Kerwat R, Shandall A, Stephenson B. Reduction of paraphimosis with granulated sugar. Br J Urol. 1998;82:755.

Kuntze JR, Lowe P, Ahlering TE. Testicular torsion after orchidopexy. J Urol. 1985;134:1209–10.

Licht MR, Montague DK, Angermeier KW, Lakin MM. Cultures from genitourinary prostheses at reoperation: questioning the role of *Staphylococcus epidermidis* in periprosthetic infection. J Urol. 1995;154:387–90.

Melloul M, Paz A, Lask D, et al. The value of radionuclide scrotal imaging in the diagnosis of acute testicular torsion. Br J Urol. 1995; 76:628–31.

Montague DK, Jarow J, Broderick GA, et al. American Urological Association guideline on the management of priapism. J Urol. 2003; 170:1318–24.

Nelson CP, Williams JF, Bloom DA. The cremasteric reflex: a useful but imperfect sign in testicular torsion. J Pediatr Surg. 2003;38: 1248–9.

Osca JM, Broseta E, Server G, et al. Unusual foreign bodies in the urethra and bladder. Br J Urol. 1991;68:510–2.

Phipps JH. Torsion of testis following orchidopexy. Br J Urol. 1987;59:596.

Reynard JM, Barua JM. Reduction of paraphimosis the simple way – the Dundee technique. Br J Urol Int. 1999;83:859–60.

Rolnick D, Kawanoue S, Szanto P, et al. Anatomical incidence of testicular appendages. J Urol. 1968;100:755.

Thurston A, Whitaker R. Torsion of testis after previous testicular surgery. Br J Surg. 1983;70:217.

van Ophoven A, de Kernion JB. Clinical management of foreign bodies of the genitourinary tract. J Urol. 2000;164:274–87.

Wallace DMA, Gunter PA, London GV, et al. Sympathetic orchidopathia, an experimental and clinical study. Br J Urol. 1982;54: 765–8.

Watkin NA, Reiger NA, Moisey CU. Conservative management of the acute scrotum. Br J Urol. 1996;78:623–7.

Further Reading

Montague DK, Angermeier KW. Artificial urinary sphincter troubleshooting. Urology. 2001;58:779–82.

Chapter 7
Postoperative Emergencies After Urological Surgery

Hashim Hashim

Shock Due To Blood Loss

Shock is defined as inadequate organ perfusion and tissue oxygenation. The causes are hypovolemia, cardiogenic, septic, anaphylactic, and neurogenic. The commonest cause of hypovolemic shock is hemorrhage. Hemorrhage is an acute loss of circulating blood volume.

Following surgery, it is important to recognize the presence of shock early, identify the cause, and treat it promptly. Hemorrhagic shock may be categorized into four classes:

1. Class I: up to 750 mL of blood loss (15% of blood volume); normal pulse rate (PR), respiratory rate (RR), blood pressure (BP), urine output, and mental status.
2. Class II: 750–1,500 mL (15–30% of blood volume), PR >100 bpm, decreased pulse pressure due to increased diastolic pressure, RR = 20–30 breaths/min, urinary output = 20–30 mL/h, mildly anxious.
3. Class III: 1,500–2,000 mL (30–40% of blood volume), PR >120 bpm, decreased blood pressure and pulse pressure due to decreased systolic pressure, RR = 30–40 breaths/min, urine output 5–15 mL/h, anxious and confused.

H. Hashim, M.D., FEBU, FRCS (Urol)
Consultant Urological Surgeon and Director of the Urodynamics Unit,
Department of Urology, Bristol Urological Institute,
Southmead Hospital, Bristol, UK
e-mail: h.hashim@gmail.com

H. Hashim et al. (eds.), *Urological Emergencies*
In Clinical Practice, DOI 10.1007/978-1-4471-2720-8_7,
© Springer-Verlag London 2013

4. Class IV: >2,000 mL (>40% of blood volume), >140 bpm, decreased pulse pressure and blood pressu.. RR >35 breaths/min, urine output <5 mL/h, lethargic. Th.. skin will feel cold and clammy.

Look at the trend in the vital signs in the hours preceding the development of shock. Examine the heart and lungs and check for capillary refill. A diagnosis of shock is based on the interpretation of clinical signs. Important parameters are the pulse rate, blood pressure, respiratory rate, urine output, and mental status. Changes in these parameters give an idea about the degree of hypoperfusion of vital organs (brain, kidneys) and therefore of the degree of bleeding.

Bleeding may be observed through a wound or drain, but the absence of blood in drains should not be taken as a sign of absent bleeding (drains can be blocked by clots). If the patient has undergone abdominal surgery, then intra-abdominal bleeding may cause abdominal distension.

Treatment

- Remember ABC (airway, breathing, and circulation). Give the patient 100% oxygen to improve tissue oxygenation.
- Perform an electrocardiogram (ECG) and put the patient on a cardiac monitor.
- Insert two short and wide intravenous (IV) cannulae in the antecubital fossa, e.g., 16G. If you cannot establish peripheral venous access due to vascular shutdown, either insert a central venous line, or perform a short saphenous vein cutdown.
- Infuse 1 L of warm Hartmann's solution, or if severe hemorrhage, then start a colloid instead, e.g., gelofusin. Aim for a urinary output of 0.5 mL/kg/h and try to maintain the blood pressure.
- Take blood samples for full blood count (FBC), coagulation screen, urea and electrolytes, and cardiac enzymes.

Cross-match six units of blood. There may already be blood in the bank, depending on the operation the patient had. Patients undergoing intermediate or major urological operations will at least have a group and save sample. If there is a delay in the arrival of the blood products, transfuse with O negative blood. You should be familiar with the location of the blood bank. It takes about 1 h to provide cross-matched blood and 10 min for type-specific blood.

- Do arterial blood gases to check for metabolic acidosis.
- If the patient does not stabilize or the situation deteriorates, then you will need to take the patient back to the operating room to stop the bleeding.

Anaphylaxis After Administration of Intravenous Contrast or Antibiotics

Anaphylaxis is usually encountered by urologists in the context of drug administration, e.g., antibiotics or following intravenous injection of an iodine-based contrast medium during intravenous urography (IVU). It is a type I hypersensitivity reaction mediated by immunoglobulin E (IgE) or IgG and the release of histamine and can lead to severe shock and death. Early recognition of its symptoms and signs is therefore very important.

Symptoms

- Itching and erythema due to urticaria and a cutaneous rash
- Shortness of breath due to angioedema or pulmonary edema
- Feeling faint and unconsciousness due to cardiovascular collapse
- Wheezing or stridor due to bronchospasm
- Abdominal pain

Signs

- Swelling of soft tissues including generalized edema, e.g., lips and eyelids
- Cyanosis
- Cold peripheries
- Pallor
- Diarrhea and vomiting

These signs and symptoms arise as a consequence of mediators of anaphylaxis acting on smooth muscle cells producing bronchospasm, vasodilation, increased capillary permeability, and secretion of exocrine glands.

Examination

- Look for soft tissue swelling
- Measure blood pressure (BP), which may be reduced
- Check the pulse for tachycardia
- Check oxygen saturation with a pulse oximeter
- Check for reduced capillary refill (>2 s) by pressing on the finger nail bed
- Listen to the chest for wheeziness, breath sounds, and heart sounds

Investigations

The diagnosis is essentially clinical.

Treatment

- Follow Advanced Life Support guidelines (ABC). Secure airway first if the patient has collapsed and start cardiac massage if pulseless.
- Stop the cause, e.g., IV infusion.
- If there is compromise to the airway, then the anesthetist needs to be called for intubation and transfer the patient to the intensive care unit (ICU).

- Administer 100% oxygen.
- Obtain IV access in the antecubital fossa with a "short and fat" venflon, e.g., 16G.
- Obtain an electrocardiogram (ECG) and place the patient on a cardiac monitor.
- Run intravenous normal saline into the drip. Use a colloid, e.g., gelofusin, if the BP has dropped.
- Administer 0.5 mL of 1:1,000 epinephrine intramuscularly (IM) or 3–5 mL of 1:10,000 epinephrine IM. Repeat every 10 min until improvement.
- If that fails, then a slow infusion of norepinephrine could be started instead, especially if 2 L of colloid have gone in without any help.
- If still no improvement, then give hydrocortisone 100 mg IV, especially if there is bronchospasm.
- If the patient has angioedema or itching, then give an anti-histamine, e.g., chlorpheniramine 10 mg IV. This can also be combined with ranitidine 50 mg IV, as a combination of H1 and H2 antagonist seems to be better.
- Other treatments that could be tried include inhaled beta-2-agonist, e.g., salbutamol 5 mg, if there is severe broncho-spasm that has not responded to other treatments.
- If the anaphylaxis is mild, then there is no need for the patient to be admitted to the ICU but will need to be observed for at least 2 h. However, if severe anaphylaxis, the patient may need inotropic support, and ICU admission will be necessary.
- Following recovery, refer patients for skin patch testing and radioimmunoassays for specific IgE to see if they are allergic to anything else. You should also explain to the patients what happened and they should carry a card with them at all times saying they have an allergy to a certain drug or contrast media.
- If they are susceptible to being exposed to the allergen, then they should be instructed to carry IM epinephrine (EpiPen) with them.

To help avoid anaphylaxis, you should always ask patients before giving them any medication or intravenous contrast, if they have any allergies at all, including drug allergies and to document that clearly in the case notes. This question should also be asked when giving the contrast intravesically, as in the case of a cystogram, although the risk of anaphylaxis is much less.

Scrotal Swelling After Scrotal Surgery

Occasionally a large scrotal hematoma can develop after scrotal surgery such as vasectomy, hydrocoele repair, or orchidectomy. This occurs in approximately 2% of cases (Kendrick et al. 1987). If the hematoma is large, surgical drainage is best carried out. It can be difficult to identify the bleeding vessel. Leave a small drain to prevent re-accumulation of the hematoma.

Wound Dehiscence Leading to Burst Abdomen

Definition

This is the disruption of the apposed surfaces of a wound resulting in the breakdown of skin and deeper musculoaponeurotic layers exposing the viscera (Dickenson and Leaper 1999). It typically occurs in the first week postoperatively (Fig. 7.1).

Factors predisposing to wound dehiscence are patient related and surgeon related. Patient-related factors include obesity, diabetes, immuno-suppression, malnutrition, malignancy, sepsis, and emergency operations. These factors favor the occurrence of wound infection and dehiscence. Other factors include coughing and straining postoperatively, which increase intra-abdominal pressure and put extra tension on the sutures.

Surgeon-related factors: tying sutures too tightly can result in the suture cutting through fascial layers. There is a higher rate of wound dehiscence where suture length is less than four times the length of the wound (Jenkins's rule).

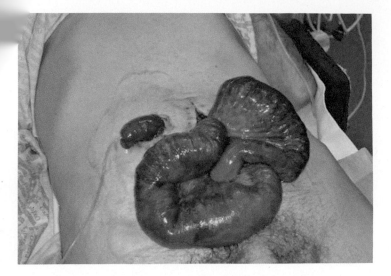

FIGURE 7.1 Burst abdomen

Diagnosis

Daily wound examination may show signs of wound infection, which predisposes to wound dehiscence. Signs of impending wound dehiscence are skin breakdown and discharge of serosanguinous "pink" fluid from the wound. You may be called to the ward because the patient's abdomen has suddenly burst, exposing the small and large bowel.

The abdominal contents should be covered with a sterile dressing, and the patient should be returned to the operating room to allow wound closure. Give intravenous analgesia, e.g., 5 mg morphine with 50 mg of intravenous cyclizine, as an antiemetic. Reassure patients and explain what has just happened and that you will need to take them back to the operating room for wound closure. At operation, wash the wound thoroughly with warm saline and debride any nonviable tissue. Re-suture the wound with interrupted, monofilament, nonabsorbable sutures. Place the sutures 1 cm apart with a fair margin from the wound edge. The size of the suture depends on the site of the wound. The key thing is to include all the layers, including peritoneum. The sutures should remain in situ for 2–3 weeks. If there is evidence of sepsis, then antibiotics should be given. In some cases, it is not possible to close the abdomen and a vacuum dressing needs to be applied and changed every 48–72 h in the operating room, which may allow the abdomen to be closed within a week.

Post-Circumcision Bleeding

Bleeding following circumcision is most likely to be from the frenular artery on the ventral surface of the penis. If local pressure does not stop the bleeding (and if it is from the frenular artery, it usually won't), take the patient to the operating room and either under penile ring block local anesthesia or general anesthetic, suture-ligated the bleeding vessel. Be careful not to place the suture through the urethra!

Not infrequently, a crust of coagulated blood develops around the circumference of the penis after circumcision. As blood oxidizes, it turns black, and this appearance can be mistaken for necrosis of the end of the penis. Reassurance of the patient (and the referring doctor!) is all that is needed.

Blocked Catheter Post-Transurethral Resection of the Prostate (TURP) and Clot Retention

In the UK National Prostatectomy Audit (Neal 1997), bleeding severe enough to require return to the operating room was reported in 0.6% of cases. Therefore, not all bleeding patients post-TURP need to return to the operating room. In many cases, the bleeding can be controlled in the recovery room or on the ward.

Cross-match blood and other blood products [platelets and fresh frozen plasma (FFP) if a large transfusion is anticipated], and give plasma expanders, if the patient shows cardiovascular compromise, while awaiting the blood.

If the catheter has blocked, take a 50-mL bladder syringe nd flush the outflow channel of the catheter (sometimes the infusion channel needs flushing to remove any clots at the end of it). Immediately aspirate urine from the outflow channel in an attempt to suck out clots contained within the bladder. Continue performing a manual bladder washout to remove any clots. If urine flow is reestablished, continue to irrigate the bladder while applying traction on the catheter so that the balloon will tamponade any bleeding vessels at the bladder neck (these may have been the source of the bleeding). Inflate the balloon of the catheter to a total of 50 mL of water (a 30-mL balloon easily accommodates this volume) to maximize this effect. Applying pressure in this way for 20 min can stop the bleeding. Traction can be applied either by you standing there or a nurse and pulling on the catheter, or hanging the bag over the end of the bed, or knotting a swab on the catheter and positioning it flush with the urethral meatus.

If bleeding continues despite traction or recurs after a period of traction, it is usually best to take the patient back to the operating room to establish where the bleeding is coming from and to control it with diathermy. This also provides the best way of removing large clots from the bladder (by using the Ellik evacuator and a large-bore resectoscope).

The same approach should be used for clot retention due to other sources of heavy hematuria. The bleeding is usually more easily controlled than with post-TURP bleeding.

Extraperitoneal Perforation During TURP

See Chap. 5.

Transurethral Resection (TUR) Syndrome

In the National Prostatectomy Audit (Neal 1997), the TUR syndrome occurred in 0.5% of cases. It is characterized by a number of symptoms and signs that may be present in

variable degree depending on the severity of the conditio
These include confusion, nausea, vomiting, hypertension, bra
dycardia, and visual disturbances.

The diagnosis of the TUR syndrome calls for a high degree
of awareness on the part of the urological team. It may be
ushered in with restlessness and hypertension and rapidly
proceed to what appears to be a grand mal seizure. If the
patient is under spinal anesthesia and is therefore awake during the procedure, he may report visual disturbances such as
flashing lights. This can be a very helpful warning that
significant amounts of glycine (and therefore fluid) are being
absorbed and that corrective measures should be started. It
does not occur if saline is used as an irrigating fluid.

One of the authors was once explaining this feature of
TUR syndrome to a junior anesthetic colleague when the
patient suddenly complained of flashing lights. The operation
was quickly brought to a conclusion, and the patient responded
rapidly to intravenous furosemide and fluid restriction, without going on to develop the more serious manifestations of
advanced TUR syndrome.

Dilutional hyponatremia is the most important and serious
factor leading to the symptoms and signs. The serum sodium
usually has to fall to below 125 mmol/L before the patient
becomes unwell. The hypertension is due to fluid overload.
Visual disturbances may be due to the fact that glycine is a
neurotransmitter in the retina.

Prevention of the TUR Syndrome

Being aware of the risk, and trying to reduce it, is the first step
to prevention. This can be achieved by using non-hemolyzing
isotonic irrigation fluids, minimizing the inflow irrigating fluid
pressure by maintaining the irrigating fluid height at 60 cm
above the symphysis pubis, using continuous flow systems to
eliminate the need for intermittent bladder evacuations, and
maintaining low fluid pressure in the prostatic fossa and bladder, with regular bladder emptying.

Any chronic hyponatremia needs to be correct preopera-tively by treating the cause and fluid restriction. Intraoperative cardiac monitoring is useful, as well as using glycine with 1% ethanol to estimate fluid absorption by monitoring ethanol excretion in expired air. If there is extensive bleeding and presumed fluid absorption occurs, then ask the anesthetist to give intravenous 0.9% saline with 20 mg of furosemide.

Definitive Treatment of TUR Syndrome

Send a sample of blood to the laboratory for serum sodium measurement and give 20–40 mg of intravenous furosemide to off-load the excess fluid that has been absorbed. In severe cases, slow administration of 200 mL of 3% hypertonic saline solution intravenously over 1–2 h may be required and repeated as necessary. This is usually done by an intensivist in the ICU. Monitor the electrolytes every 2–4 h to prevent over-correction. Patients usually become asymptomatic by increasing sodium by 4–6 mmol/L. Rarely is hemodialysis required.

No more than half the expected sodium deficit needs correcting in the first 24 h and no more than half of this amount should be corrected with hypertonic saline. Replacement should be done slowly. Avoid an increase in sodium by more than 20 mmol/L over 24 h. Ideally, correct at no more than 0.5 mmol/L/h.

The amount of saline required to replace the deficit is the estimated total sodium deficit divided by the sodium content of the replacement fluid.

$$[\textbf{Na deficit} = (\text{Desired target} - \text{Serum Na}) \times (\text{Body weight in kg} \times 0.6)]$$

- 0.9% Saline = 154 mmol/L Na
- 3% Saline = 513 mmol/L Na

Displaced Catheter
Post-radical Prostatectomy

Urethral catheters are left in situ post-radical prostatectomy for a variable time depending on the surgeon who performs the operation. Some surgeons leave a catheter for 3 weeks and others for just 1 week. Thus, if a catheter falls out a week after surgery, the patient may well void successfully, and in this situation, no further action needs be taken.

If, however, the catheter inadvertently falls out the day after surgery, we would make a gentle attempt to replace it with a 12 Fr catheter that has been well lubricated. If this fails, we would pass a flexible cystoscope, under local anesthetic, into the bulbar urethra and attempt to pass a guidewire into the bladder, over which a catheter can then safely be passed. If this is not possible, another option is to hope that the patient voids spontaneously and does not leak urine at the site of the anastomosis. An ascending urethrogram may provide reassurance that there is no leak of contrast and that the anastomosis is watertight. If there is a leak or the patient is unable to void, a suprapubic catheter could be placed, either percutaneously (ultrasound guidance may be needed) or under general anesthetic via an open cystostomy.

The same principles would apply if the patient had an orthotopic neobladder formation or an artificial urinary sphincter inserted.

Compartment Syndrome of the Lower Limb Associated with the Lithotomy Position

Lower limb compartment syndrome (LLCS) is the development of an increased tissue pressure within the closed osteofascial compartment of the leg, which reduces perfusion of the leg leading to ischemia of the muscles and nerves. If prolonged, it leads to permanent loss of function in the affected muscles and nerves. In the context of urological surgery, LLCS is specifically associated with the lithotomy position and is said to occur with a frequency in the order of 1 in 3,500 (Halliwell et al. 1998). Thus, it is rare, but because the consequences of missing the diagnosis of LLCS are devastating, it is important to appreciate its predisposing factors, presentation, and subsequent management.

The leg has four osteofascial compartments, which are bordered by nonelastic fascia and bone. Normal resting tissue pressure in the anterior compartment of the leg ranges between 3 and 22 mmHg.

Mechanisms

Any factor that induces ischemia in the leg can lead to a compartment syndrome. Ischemia disrupts the integrity of the vascular endothelium, leading to fluid shifts into the extracellular tissue space with a consequent rise in tissue pressure. The lithotomy position causes ischemia in the leg by the following mechanisms:

1. Reduction in hydrostatic perfusion pressure. Every 1-cm elevation of the limb above the heart reduces mean arteriolar pressure by 1 mmHg and causes a measurable reduction in ankle–brachial pressure index. This reduction in perfusion pressure is compounded by the head-down position
2. Calf compression. This can occlude both venous drainage and arterial flow.
3. Knee and hip flexion can compress blood vessels.
4. Dorsiflexion of the foot causes an increase in pressure within the calf.

As compartment pressure rises, the lumen of arterioles is eventually occluded. A vicious cycle of ischemia sets in. When the limb is returned to the supine position, a reperfusion injury can cause a further rise in compartment pressure.

The major factor determining the likelihood of development of a LLCS is time spent in the lithotomy position. The exaggerated lithotomy position is more likely to lead to a LLCS than is a lower lithotomy position. Hypotension, hypovolemia, and peripheral vascular disease, all predispose to development of the compartment syndrome. Young, large men with an increased muscle bulk may be at greater risk of a compartment syndrome because of tighter, less compliant compartments in the leg.

Presentation and Treatment

The classic presentation is with pain in the leg and paresthesia. Passive stretching of the affected muscles causes worsening of the pain. The pain may be out of all proportion to the physical signs. The skin may be pink, and the pulse may still be present. It is possible to measure compartment pressures, but the equipment for doing this, and expertise in recording and interpreting the pressures measured, is unlikely to be available in many cases. A high index of suspicion, therefore, is required to make a clinical diagnosis.

The mainstay of treatment is decompression of the affected compartment by a fasciotomy. Ideally such a procedure should be carried out by an expert (orthopedic, vascular, or plastic surgeon), but if this is unlikely to be available at very short notice, the urologist will have to proceed with fasciotomy, relying on his anatomical knowledge to avoid damage to structures such as the common peroneal nerve.

Metabolic Complications

Hypercalcemia

Hypercalcemia may be a manifestation of a variety of disorders including hyperparathyroidism, sarcoidosis, multiple myeloma, hyperthyroidism, acute osteoporosis, metastatic bone disease, and a number of primary malignancies. The neoplasms most commonly associated with hypercalcemia include carcinoma of the lung (all cell types), breast cancer, squamous cell carcinomas, hematologic malignancies, and renal cell carcinoma. 90% of hypercalcemia is due to primary

erparathyroidism or malignancy. Normal serum calcium
vels are 2.2–2.6 mmol/L (9–10.5 mg/dL).

Patient's symptoms can be remembered by the phrase,
"stones, bones, groans, thrones, and psychiatric overtones."
Therefore patients can present with renal or biliary stones,
bone pain, abdominal pain, nausea and vomiting, sit on the
throne (polyuria), depression (30–40%), anxiety, cognitive
dysfunction, insomnia, and coma, as well as malaise and
fatigue. Electrocardiogram (ECG) changes include a short
QT interval and widened T waves.

The initial treatment involves reducing serum calcium
levels and increasing urinary calcium excretion followed by
treating the underlying cause if possible. Initial treatment is
achieved by adequate oral or intravenous hydration with
0.9% normal saline. Addition of a loop diuretic, such as furosemide, will also help in reducing reabsorption and increasing excretion of calcium, as well as preventing overhydration.
Patients in renal failure may require dialysis. These measures can usually decrease serum calcium by 1–3 mg/dL
within 24 h.

If the above fail to reduce calcium levels then an intravenous infusion of bisphosphonates, such as pamidronate or
zoledronate, is given. These agents inhibit osteoclastic bone
resorption. If these fail then calcitonin, a naturally occurring
hormone that inhibits bone reabsorption, and increases
excretion of calcium, can be given. The effects of calcitonin
may be observed within a few hours with peak response at
12–24 h.

Hypocalcemia

This can occur in acute renal failure or parathyroid hormone
deficiency. Symptoms include convulsions, arrhythmias, tet-
any, and numbness/paresthesia in the hands, feet, around the
mouth, and lips.

Treatment in the acute setting includes 10 mL of 10%
intravenous calcium gluconate slowly over a period of 10 min,
or if severe, then calcium chloride can be given instead. It is

important not to give this via a drip that has been used sodium bicarbonate infusion, as insoluble calcium carbon (chalk) will form. Also, this regime is only for acute hypoca cemia over a short period of time.

Hyperkalemia

This may be caused by the ineffective elimination of potassium, excessive release from cells or excessive intake. Causes include renal failure due to outlet obstruction causing high pressure urinary retention, metabolic acidosis, potassium sparing diuretics, rhabdomyolysis, burns, metabolic acidosis, excess potassium supplements, Addison's disease, and medications such as angiotensin converting enzyme inhibitors.

Symptoms are fairly vague and may include malaise, palpitations, and muscle weakness. Hyperkalemia can lead to cardiac arrest if levels are above 6.5 mmol/L (normal levels: 3.5–5 mmol/L). Diagnosis is made on blood testing. An ECG can show tall tented T waves (gothic T waves), small P wave, increased P-R interval, and wide QRS complex (sine wave).

Treatment is indicated if there are cardiac arrhythmias or potassium levels are above 6.5 mmol/L. This includes treating the cause, e.g., catheterizing a patient who has renal failure secondary to prostatic obstruction.

Calcium gluconate is given (10 mL of 10% intravenously over 2 min) and is cardioprotective. Onset of action is within 5 min and lasts about 30–60 min. There should be constant ECG monitoring, and the dose repeated if no response is seen on ECG.

Insulin is given intravenously, to increase cellular potassium uptake, with dextrose, to prevent hypoglycemia: 10-mL soluble insulin in 50-mL 50% dextrose over 5 min. This lowers potassium levels within 20 min, and effects last up to 6 h. This can be supplemented with a salbutamol (β2-agonist) nebulizer (5 mg) and bicarbonate (1 ampoule (50 mEq) infused over 5 min). In acute renal failure, high-dose furosemide may be required (250 mg intravenously over 5 min), and in severe cases, hemodialysis or filtration may be needed.

abolic Acidosis

his condition occurs when the body produces too much acid or when the kidneys are not removing enough acid from the body. In urology, it occurs usually when a segment of bowel is used in urinary tract reconstruction.

Symptoms are rather nonspecific, and therefore it needs to be on the differential diagnosis of patients who have had urinary reconstruction using a bowel segment. Symptoms develop over time and could include anorexia, weight loss, polydipsia, lethargy, and easy fatigability. Others could include chest pain, palpitation, headache, altered mental status such as severe anxiety due to hypoxia, decreased visual acuity, nausea, vomiting, abdominal pain, altered appetite, muscle weakness, and bone pains.

If small bowel or colon were used in the reconstruction, then patients could develop hyperchloremic metabolic acidosis, and if stomach is used, then they can develop hypochloremic metabolic acidosis.

Diagnosis is made with arterial blood gas sampling where the pH will be low (<7.35). The base excess may be less than −3 mmol/L. Venous blood sampling for electrolytes, bicarbonate (low <20 mmol/L), chloride, renal function, full blood count, and glucose are all important. Urinalysis by dipstick testing is important to look for acidity/alkalinity and ketones. Calculate the anion gap $[(Na^+ + K^+) - (Cl^- + HCO_3^-)]$ which should be normal (<20) in urinary diversion cases.

Treatment is based on correction of the acidosis with sodium bicarbonate tablets (500 mg three times per day) initially if the patient can be treated on an outpatient basis. If the pH is less than 7.1, then the patient needs admission and possibly treated with intravenous hypertonic sodium bicarbonate (two 50-mL ampoules of 8.4% $NaHCO_3$ (containing 50 mEq each)) under strict arterial blood gas monitoring in liaison with the nephrologists and intensivists in a high dependency unit/ICU. The patient may require dialysis. If there is hypokalemia then potassium citrate can be used.

References

Dickenson AJ, Leaper DJ. Wound dehiscence and incisional hern
Surgery. 1999;17:229–32.

Halliwell JR, Hewitt BS, Joyner MH, Warner MA. Effect of various
lithotomy positions on lower extremity pressure. Anesthesiology.
1998;89:1373–6.

Kendrick J, Gonzales B, Huber D, et al. Complications of vasecto-
mies in the United States. J Fam Pract. 1987,25:245–8.

Neal DE. The national prostatectomy audit. Br J Urol. 1997;79
Suppl 2.69–75.

Further Reading

American College of Surgeons Committee on Trauma. Advanced
trauma life support for doctors—student course manual. 6th ed.
Chicago: American College of Surgeons; 1999.

Webb A, Shapiro M, Singer M, et al. Oxford textbook of critical care.
Oxford: Oxford Medical Publications; 1999.

Chapter 8
Ureteric Colic in Pregnancy

Dan Wood

The incidence of ureteric colic is probably unchanged by pregnancy, ranging from 1 in 1,500 to 1 in 2,500 – the same as in nonpregnant women (Coe et al. 1978). Some authors have suggested the incidence increases significantly up to 1 in 200 (Cormier et al. 2006), although evidence to support this is limited. Ureteric colic in pregnant women tends to occur during the second or third trimester (Stothers and Lee 1992). Both urinary calcium and uric acid excretion increase in pregnancy (predisposing to stone formation), so too do urinary citrate and magnesium levels (protecting against stone formation). The development of a ureteric stone during pregnancy is a significant event for four important reasons:

- Pain and the challenge of providing safe analgesia in pregnancy.
- Difficulty with providing a safe and effective diagnostic modality.

D. Wood, Ph.D., FRCS (Urol)
Department of Adolescent and Reconstructive Urology,
University College London Hospitals,
London, UK

Department of Urology, Great Ormond Street Hospital,
London, UK

University College London,
London, UK
e-mail: dan.wood@uclh.nhs.uk

H. Hashim et al. (eds.), *Urological Emergencies In Clinical Practice*, DOI 10.1007/978-1-4471-2720-8_8, © Springer-Verlag London 2013

223

- Safe and effective treatment can be difficult.
- Increased risk of early labor (Hendricks et al. 1991)

The Hydronephrosis of Pregnancy

In 90 % of pregnancies the kidneys are hydronephrotic, and this develops from approximately week 6 to week 10 of gestation. Resolution is usually complete within 2 months of delivery (Peake et al. 1983). Hydronephrosis during pregnancy is thought to occur due to a combined smooth muscle relaxant effect of progesterone and mechanical obstruction from a gravid uterus (Chaliha and Stanton 2002). Hydronephrosis is said not to occur in pelvic kidneys, nor does it occur in quadripeds such as dogs and cats where the uterus is dependent and thus "falls" away from the ureter (Robert 1976). Patients who have undergone previous reconstruction of the urinary tract need closer monitoring as their risk of hydronephrosis appears to be greater and intervention may be necessary in up to 10 % (Greenwell et al. 2003) – principles of diagnosis and management are similar to those below, but for those with symptoms or earlier than expected hydronephrosis, monthly ultrasounds are a useful means of surveillance with percutaneous nephrostomy (rather than retrograde stent) being the preferred method of drainage.

Hydronephrosis associated with flank pain in a pregnant lady poses a diagnostic dilemma. The desire to avoid using ionizing radiation in pregnant women needs to be balanced against the limitations of other forms of imaging. Renal ultrasonography is often used as the initial imaging technique in those presenting with flank pain – this is a view supported within the EAU guidelines, but its limitations are acknowledged (Türk et al. 2012). In the nonpregnant patient, the presence of hydronephrosis may be taken as surrogate evidence of ureteric obstruction. Because hydronephrosis is a normal finding in the majority of pregnancies, its presence is an unreliable sign of a possible

eric stone. In a series of pregnant women, ultrasound
d a sensitivity of 34 % (i.e., it misses 66 % of stones) and
specificity of 86 % for detecting an abnormality in the
presence of a stone (i.e., false-positive rate of 14 %)
(Stothers and Lee 1992).

Presentation of Stones in Pregnancy

Flank pain remains the usual presentation, with or without
hematuria (macroscopic or microscopic). Differential diagnoses include urinary tract infection, placental abruption, or
appendicitis.

What Imaging Study Should Be Used to Establish Diagnosis of a Ureteric Stone in Pregnancy?

Exposure of a fetus to ionizing radiation raises concerns
about fetal malformations, malignancies in later life (leukemia), and mutagenic effects (damage to genes causing inher-
ited disease in the offspring of the fetus). The risk to the fetus
is highest in the first trimester. Fetal radiation doses during
various procedures are shown in Table 8.1.

TABLE 8.1 Fetal radiation doses after various radiological
investigations

Procedure	Mean fetal dose mGy	Risk of inducing cancer up to age 15 years
KUB X-ray	1.4	–
IVU 6 shot	1.7	1 in 10,000
CT-abdominal	8	–
CT-pelvic	25	–
Fluoroscopy for JJ stent insertion	0.4	1 in 42,000

Radiation doses of <100 mGy are very unlikely to have adverse effect on the fetus (Hellawell et al. 2002). In USA, the National Council on Radiation Protection (NCR. has stated, "Fetal risk is considered to be negligible a. <50 mGy when compared to the other risks of pregnancy, and the risk of malformations is significantly increased above control levels at doses >150 mGy" (NCRP 1997). The American College of Obstetricians and Gynecologists (ACOG) has stated, "X-ray exposure to <50 mGy has not been associated with an increase in fetal anomalies or pregnancy loss" (ACOG 1995).

While these recommended maximum radiation levels are well above those occurring even during computed tomography (CT) scanning, and a dose of 50 mGy or less is regarded as safe, there remains a concern that any radiation dose exposes the fetus to some risk. For this reason, every effort should be made to limit exposure of the fetus to ionizing radiation and to find an alternative where possible. However, the pregnant woman may be reassured that the likely risk to her unborn child as a consequence of radiation exposure is minimal.

Investigations or treatments that involve exposure to ionizing radiation should not be withheld because of an unjustified fear of damaging the fetus. The risks for the fetus have to be balanced against the risks of missing the diagnosis of a stone obstructing the ureter and the difficulties and potential dangers of performing a percutaneous nephrostomy, JJ stent insertion, or ureteroscopy without the use of any (ionizing radiation) imaging.

Plain Radiography and Intravenous Urography (IVU)

These studies have limitations in pregnancy. First, the fetal skeleton and the enlarged uterus may obscure ureteric stones, so the imaging study may not be diagnostic. Second, there may be delayed excretion of contrast as a consequence of the physiological dilatation of the kidney. It can be difficult, if not

possible, to differentiate this "physiological" delay from
at due to an obstructing stone. Third, there is also the
neoretical risk of fetal toxicity from the contrast media,
though none has been reported.

Ultrasound

Ultrasound is an unreliable way of diagnosing the presence
of stones in pregnant women. Jets of urine expelled by normal peristalsis of the nonobstructed ureter can be seen on
ultrasound scanning (Fig. 8.1), and the absence of such ureteric jets is said to have a high sensitivity and specificity for
diagnosing obstructing stones (Doyle et al. 1995), though others have reported that ureteric jets may be absent in an
asymptomatic pregnant women (Burke and Washowich 1998).

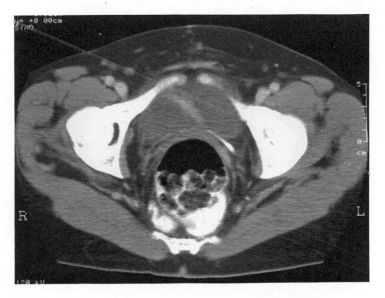

FIGURE 8.1 Jets of urine expelled by normal peristalsis of the nonobstructed ureter can be seen on ultrasound scanning or on computed tomography (CT) (as shown here). CT should be avoided if at
all possible in pregnancy

It is very important to understand these limitations, ultrasound remains the recommended first line for diagnos of urolithiasis in pregnancy. The addition of a transvagina scan may improve visualization of the lower ureters (Türk et al. 2012).

Computed Tomography Urography (CTU)

Although CT urography is a very accurate method for detecting ureteric stones and the radiation dose is below 50 mGy, most radiologists and urologists do not recommend this form of imaging in pregnant women. Magnetic resonance urography (see below) provides an alternative form of imaging in this difficult group of patients.

Magnetic Resonance Urography (MRU)

The American College of Obstetricians and Gynecologists and the U.S. National Council on Radiation Protection state, "Although there is no evidence to suggest that the embryo is sensitive to magnetic and radiofrequency at the intensities encountered in MRI, it might be prudent to exclude pregnant women during the first trimester" (ACOG 1995; NCRP 1997). Given this advice, therefore, MRU can potentially be used during the second and third trimesters, but not during the first trimester.

MRU avoids ionizing radiation and can be done with the administration of contrast (Fig. 8.2). It can be accurate, with one group reporting sensitivity for detecting ureteric stones of 100 % (Roy et al. 1996). However, MRU is expensive and not readily available in all hospitals, particularly out of hours – the stone is generally seen as a filling defect, thus the findings are not specific. As MR scanners become more widespread, it is likely that this imaging modality will be used increasingly to establish a diagnosis in pregnant women with flank pain (Bott et al. 2012).

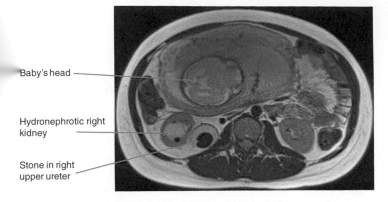

Baby's head

Hydronephrotic right kidney

Stone in right upper ureter

FIGURE 8.2 MRI scan demonstrating the foetus and the stone in the right upper ureter

Management of Ureteric Stones in Pregnant Women

The majority (70–80 %) of ureteric stones in pregnant women will pass spontaneously (Stothers and Lee 1992). On this basis, conservative management is recommended as the first line of treatment. Of those that do not and require temporizing treatment with nephrostomy tube drainage or JJ stents, many will pass without further intervention. Opiate-based analgesics are used for pain relief and oral and intravenous fluids for hydration. Nonsteroidal anti-inflammatory drugs (NSAIDs) should be avoided because they can cause premature closure of the ductus arteriosus by blocking prostaglandin synthesis.

The indications for intervention are similar to those in nonpregnant patients and include pain refractory to analgesics, suspected urinary sepsis (high fever, high white count), high-grade obstruction, and obstruction in a solitary kidney.

Options for intervention are insertion of a JJ urinary stent, percutaneous nephrostomy, or ureteroscopic stone removal. The final choice of treatment will depend on the stage of pregnancy, local facilities, and expertise. Management cases requiring active intervention should aim to minimi radiation exposure to the fetus and to minimize the risk c miscarriage and preterm labor. While ureteroscopy can be performed without fluoroscopy (Rittenberg and Bagley 1988), most urologists nowadays perform the majority of their ureteroscopic work under fluoroscopic control, and in such a case that is already high risk, will be uncomfortable in compromising available information. It is worth remembering that the radiation dose during fluoroscopy for JJ stent placement is very low (approximately 0.4 mGy, and up to a maximum of 0.8 mGy) and that the dose used to assist ureteroscopy is likely to be little more than this.

General anesthesia carries a small risk of triggering a preterm labor (Duncan et al. 1986), and with this in mind, many urologists and obstetricians use a nephrostomy tube drainage or JJ stent placement, as first-line treatment, rather than ureteroscopic stone removal.

Percutaneous nephrostomy insertion diverts urine out through a silicone tube – usually inserted in the flank region; it has the advantage of being possible under local anesthetic and sedation avoiding a general anesthetic. It is widely available (Fig. 8.3), can be done rapidly, provides good pain relief, drains infected urine (if present), and has a low risk of inducing miscarriage or preterm labor (Kavoussi et al. 1992). These advantages must be weighed against the fact that there is a small risk (in the order of 1 %) of heavy bleeding, requiring embolization and/or blood transfusion during nephrostomy insertion, and of septicemic shock occurring after insertion (2–4 %; Ho et al. 2002; Ramchandani et al. 2001) (see Chap. 11). Furthermore, the nephrostomy tube may be required for some months, particularly when it is inserted at a relatively early stage in the pregnancy – a series of planned changes will need to be arranged, we would do this at 6 weekly intervals – though this is arguable, we would rather avoid the need for a second puncture. The tube can be uncomfortable, it may still block or become infected, and may need to be changed several times during the remaining pregnancy.

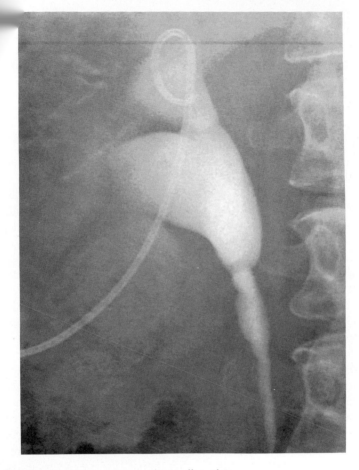

FIGURE 8.3 Nephrostomy urinary diversion

JJ stents overcome some of the problems of nephrostomy tube drainage. They can also be placed under local anesthetic or with light sedation with low doses of pethidine and diazemuls using either ultrasound guidance or limited periods of fluoroscopy (Hellawell et al. 2002; (Stothers and Lee 1992) (see Chap. 11).

A stent is an effective way of managing the pain caused obstructing stones. They may be more comfortable than pe_ cutaneous tube drainage, though many patients develop "stent symptoms" (frequency, urgency, and bladder pain), which can be so bothersome that in some cases the stent has to be removed (Hellawell et al. 2002).

In two series totaling 20 pregnant women who underwent JJ stent placement (all under local anesthetic or with sedo-analgesia), at between 6 and 36 weeks' gestation (mean 31 weeks), there were no cases of premature labor (Hellawell et al. 2002; Stothers and Lee 1992).

The hypercalciuria of pregnancy may make stent encrustation and blockage more likely, and as a consequence, it has been suggested that stents should be changed every 6–8 weeks to prevent the occurrence of blockage from encrustation (Kavoussi et al. 1992). However, in a contemporary series where stent insertion was performed at an average of 28 weeks of gestation for obstructing ureteric stones, stent replacement was not required in any patient (Hellawell et al. 2002), and in a slightly older series, only 1 of 13 stents required replacement because of ongoing pain (presumably indicating obstruction) (Stothers and Lee 1992). It may well be, therefore, that regular stent changes, at least when using contemporary stents, are not required. Avoiding the need to change JJ stents is clearly desirable, as this is technically more challenging than replacing a percutaneous nephrostomy tube (though the difficulty of placement and replacement depend on the availability of local expertise). Therefore, one might be more inclined to recommend a nephrostomy tube, rather than a JJ stent, in very early pregnancy to minimize the impact of further changes (Denstedt and Razvi 1992). Should the nephrostomy become a problem, it also offers the flexibility to convert to a stent by antegrade insertion – the reverse is not true.

JJ stents have been reported to become obstructed by mechanical impingement of the fetal head (Hellawell et al. 2002), and they may migrate down the ureter and into the bladder and subsequently be voided per urethra as a consequence of the dilatation of the ureter that is normally a feature of pregnancy (Stothers and Lee 1992).

ureteroscopic stone extraction can be performed in pregnancy, but its use depends on available expertise. Distortion of the distal third of the ureter during the latter stages of pregnancy makes rigid ureteroscopy technically challenging, as does the presence of a large stone. For these reasons the less experienced ureteroscopist may decide that nephrostomy tube drainage or a JJ stent is a better option later on in pregnancy, with subsequent ureteroscopic treatment being used if the stone fails to pass within a few weeks of delivery. In solitary kidneys, nephrostomy tube drainage or a JJ stent may also be safer options rather than attempting ureteroscopic stone extraction under the difficult conditions of late pregnancy.

References

American College of Obstetricians and Gynecologists Committee on Obstetric Practice. Guidelines for diagnostic imaging during pregnancy. ACOG Committee Opinion No. 158. Washington DC: ACOG; 1995.

Bott S, Patel U, Djavan B, Carroll P. Images in urology. Diagnosis and management. London: Springer; 2012.

Burke BJ, Washowich TL. Ureteral jets in normal second- and third trimester pregnancy. J Clin Ultrasound. 1998;26:423–6.

Chaliha C, Stanton SL. Urological problems in pregnancy. BJU Int. 2002;89:469–76.

Coe FL, Parks JH, Lindhermer MD. Nephrolithiasis during pregnancy. N Engl J Med. 1978;298:324–6.

Cormier CM, Canzoneri BJ, Lewis DF, Briery C, Knoepp L, Mailhes JB. Urolithiasis in pregnancy: current diagnosis, treatment, and pregnancy complications. Obstet Gynecol Surv. 2006;61(11): 733–41.

Denstedt JD, Razvi H. Management of urinary calculi during pregnancy. J Urol. 1992;148:1072–5.

Doyle LA, Cronan JJ, Breslaw BH, Ridlen MS. New techniques of ultrasound and color Doppler in the prospective evaluation of acute renal obstruction: do they replace the intravenous urogram? Abdom Imaging. 1995;20:58–63.

Duncan PG, Pope WD, Cohen MM, Green N. Fetal risk of anesth▮ and surgery during pregnancy. Anesthesiology. 1986;64:790–4.

Greenwell TJ, Venn SN, Creighton S, Leaver RB, Woodhouse CR▮ Pregnancy after lower urinary tract reconstruction for congenital anomalies. BJU Int. 2003;92:773–7.

Hellawell GO, Cowan NC, Holt SJ, Mutch SJ. A radiation perspective for treating loin pain in pregnancy by double-pigtail stents. BJU Int. 2002;90:801–8.

Hendricks SK, Ross SO, Krieger JN. An algorithm for diagnosis and therapy of management and complications of urolithiasis during pregnancy. Surg Gynecol Obstet. 1991;172:49–54.

Ho S, Cowan NC, Holt SJ, et al. Percutaneous nephrostomy (PCN): preliminary results from a prospective pilot study. Eur J Radiol. 2002;12:D3.

Kavoussi LR, Albala DM, Basler JW, et al. Percutaneous management of urolithiasis during pregnancy. J Urol. 1992;148:1069–71.

National Council on Radiation Protection and Measurement. Medical radiation exposure of pregnant and potentially pregnant women. NCRP report no. 54. Bethesda: NCRPM; 1997.

Peake SL, Rowburgh HB, Le Planglois S. Ultrasonic assessment of hydronephrosis in pregnancy. Radiology. 1983;146:167–70.

Ramchandani P, et al. Quality improvement guidelines for percutaneous nephrostomy. J Vasc Interv Radiol. 2001;12:1247–51.

Rittenberg MH, Bagley DH. Ureteroscopic diagnosis and treatment of urinary calculi during pregnancy. Urology. 1988;32:427–8.

Robert JA. Hydronephrosis of pregnancy. Urology. 1976;8:1–4.

Roy C, Saussine C, Le Bras Y, et al. Assessment of painful ureterohydronephrosis during pregnancy by MR urography. Eur Radiol. 1996;6:334–8.

Stothers L, Lee LM. Renal colic in pregnancy. J Urol. 1992;148:1383–7.

Türk C, Knoll T, Petrik A, Sarica K, Straub M, Seitz C. Guidelines on urolithiasis, vol. 16. Arnhem: European Association of Urology; 2012. ISBN 90806179-3-8.

Chapter 9
Management of Urological Neoplastic Conditions Presenting as Emergencies

Dan Wood

Testicular Cancer

Approximately 10 % of cases of testicular cancer present with metastatic disease – the most common sites are retroperitoneum (retroperitoneal node involvement causing back pain), chest (breathlessness, cough), and neck (enlarged cervical nodes, tracheal compression, and deviation). Spread to the central nervous system or involvement of peripheral nerves can result in neurological manifestations (Fig. 9.1). While most such cases present directly to oncologists, from time to time the urologist is the first port of call. Such cases should be referred to the oncologists as a matter of urgency for high-dose chemotherapy.

D. Wood, Ph.D., FRCS (Urol)
Department of Adolescent and Reconstructive Urology,
University College London Hospitals,
London, UK

Department of Urology, Great Ormond Street Hospital,
London, UK

University College London,
London, UK
e-mail: dan.wood@uclh.nhs.uk

H. Hashim et al. (eds.), *Urological Emergencies*
In Clinical Practice, DOI 10.1007/978-1-4471-2720-8_9,
© Springer-Verlag London 2013

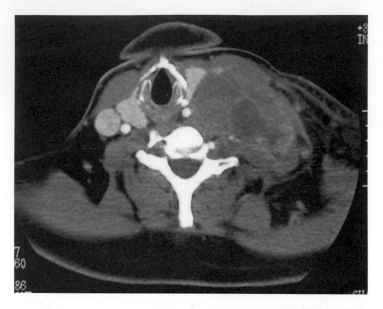

FIGURE 9.1 Advanced testicular malignancy with nodal metastases in the neck causing tracheal deviation

Malignant Ureteric Obstruction

Any of the major pelvic malignancies, prostate (in men) (Clarke 2003), cervical (in women), bladder, and rectal, may present with renal failure secondary to ureteric obstruction (Soper et al. 1988). The anatomy demonstrated in Fig. 9.2 illustrates why this is so for urological malignancies.

Other malignancies (colon, stomach, lymphoma, breast, bronchus) may metastasize to pelvic and retroperitoneal lymph nodes, causing unilateral or bilateral malignant ureteric obstruction. In unilateral obstruction with a normally functioning contralateral kidney, the obstruction proceeds silently. In bilateral obstruction, oliguria followed by anuria, and finally renal failure, is the mode of presentation.

The emergency presentation is usually one of a patient with acute renal failure, who may or may not be known to have cancer. Patients present with a rising creatinine and symptoms

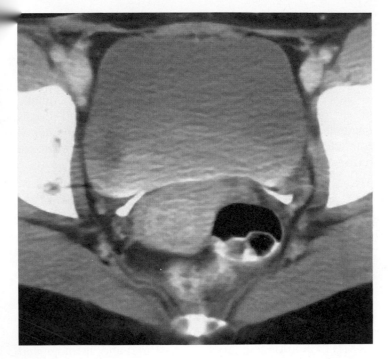

FIGURE 9.2 A computed tomography (CT) scan of the bladder showing the ureters entering posteriorly (outlined with contrast). The ureters enter the bladder just a few centimeters from the bladder neck
and can easily be obstructed by locally advanced prostate cancer

of renal failure including malaise, nausea, vomiting, and in
some cases marked oliguria or anuria as the locally advanced
or nodal metastases obstruct their ureters. This presentation is
sometimes mistaken for urinary retention, particularly if the
patient has some lower abdominal pain. However, when the
bladder is scanned or catheterized only a small volume of
urine is demonstrated, and the high creatinine level does not
fall following catheterization. In the case of prostate cancer,
digital rectal examination (DRE) reveals a firm (craggy) prostate that has extended laterally. A locally advanced rectal
cancer may be felt on DRE, and in women vaginal examination may reveal a hard, craggy mass arising from the cervix.

Clinical examination should include a DRE in both men and women. Vaginal and breast examination should be performed in women. General examination may reveal other evidence of malignant disease such as cachexia, abdominal masses, ascites, or skin nodules. Lymphandenopathy, including cervical and axillary, needs to be looked for. Measure the serum creatinine as part of a routine blood screen. A renal ultrasound reveals bilateral hydronephrosis, with an empty bladder. An abdominal computed tomography (CT) scan may demonstrate evidence of retroperitoneal and pelvic lymphadenopathy.

Emergency Treatment

In cases of prostate cancer, high-dose dexamethasone has been shown to result in an improvement in urine output and reduction in serum creatinine within 24–48 h (Hamdy and Williams 1995). Give an 8-mg intravenous (IV) bolus followed by 4 mg IV every 6 h for 3 days, switching to oral dexamethasone thereafter. A reducing regimen can be used over the course of the next month. All cases should be discussed at an MDT (multidisciplinary team meeting) and oncology and palliative care teams involved as appropriate.

Where the patient is uremic or has a rising serum potassium, more urgent treatment may be required. A percutaneous nephrostomy tube is an option, or if the patient is too unwell for this, acute hemodialysis.

In our experience, attempts at retrograde JJ stent placement in the acute situation can be very difficult and often fail (it is impossible to pass a guidewire past the area of ureteric obstruction). A nephrostomy tube allows subsequent antegrade JJ stenting, and this may become the definitive management method, with the stents being changed every few months. In the case of prostate cancer, hormone treatment should be started (if not already done so) in the form of emergency orchidectomy or with antiandrogen blockade followed by a luteinizing hormone-releasing hormone (LHRH) agonist. LHRH antagonists may also be useful in these cases instead of using an antiandrogen with an LHRH agonist.

There are clearly issues related to the long-term prognosis of such patients. Patients with cervical and prostate cancer can survive for many months after presenting with ureteric obstruction, whereas the prognosis in patients with ureteric obstruction due to other cancers tends to be considerably shorter. Fallon and colleagues (1980) reported a median survival in prostate cancer patients treated with nephrostomy drainage for bilateral ureteric obstruction of 7 months post-nephrostomy insertion, and 55 % of patients survived for over 1 year. For cervical cancer patients, the average survival was 18 months. Bladder cancer patients did poorly, with a median survival of just 4 months after nephrostomy drainage.

Spinal Cord Compression in Patients with Urological Disease

Cord compression is an uncommon presentation in patients with malignant disease; however, it does need to be considered and can be missed. Failure to diagnose and treat cord compression can have a devastating impact on quality of life. Urologists should be aware of the presentation and management of cord compression, particularly since prostate cancer is the second most common cause of malignant spinal cord compression. Local extension of a vertebral metastasis compresses the spinal cord, leading to venous obstruction and edema (at this stage, steroids can decrease the edema and reverse the neurological symptoms and prevent further progression). The majority of cases involve the thoracic or lumbar spine; the cervical spine is infrequently involved.

All too often patients with spinal cord compression have warning symptoms and signs, the significance of which is not appreciated until irreversible damage to the spinal cord has occurred. Patients are then condemned to spend their remaining months of life in a wheelchair. In a review of 24 patients presenting with cord compression due to metastatic prostate cancer (Tazi et al. 2003), 79 % had thoracic or lumbar back pain severe enough to require opiate pain relief, on average for 60 days (and ranging from 10 to 840 days) before they finally presented with neurological symptoms such as paralysis. Occasionally, cord compression is the first presenting event in a patient with metastatic prostate cancer.

Back pain is the most common early presenting symptom. It is usually gradual in onset and progresses slowly but relentlessly. The pain may be localized to the area of vertebral metastasis, but may also involve adjacent spinal nerve roots, causing radicular pain. Interscapular pain that wakes the patient at night is a characteristic of a metastatic deposit. Associated symptoms suggestive of a neurological cause for the pain include pins and needles, weakness in the arms (cervical cord) or legs (lumbosacral spine), urinary symptoms such as hesitancy and a poor urinary flow, constipation, loss of erections, and seemingly bizarre symptoms such as loss of sensation of orgasm or absent ejaculation. From time to time the patient may present in urinary retention – this is typically painless. It is all too easy to assume that this is due to malignant prostatic obstruction if other neurological symptoms and signs are not sought.

The physical sign of spinal cord compression is a sensory level, but this tends to occur late in the course of cord compression. Perform a digital rectal examination. There may be decreased sensation over the genitalia and around the anus with decreased anal tone and squeeze. If the bladder is distended, then you will need to pass a urethral catheter. Ask the patient if he/she can feel the catheter going through the urethra and into the bladder. If they have cauda equine, then they would have lost that sensation. If the sensation is present, it does not rule out cauda equine. Remember, however, that a normal neurological examination does not exclude a diagnosis of cord compression. If on the basis of the patient's symptoms you suspect cord compression, arrange for a magnetic resonance imaging (MRI) without delay.

Imaging in Suspected Cord Compression

While plain X-rays of the cervical, thoracic, and lumbar spine can show vertebral metastases in over 80 % of symptomatic patients, MRI allows accurate identification and localization of metastases and is the imaging modality of choice.

Treatment

This is a frightening and potentially devastating set of symptoms – it is very important to explain what is happening to the patient, as things may happen quickly.

In the majority of patients, initial treatment consists of pain relief, corticosteroids, and androgen deprivation (if not already started), followed by radiotherapy. Catheterization is important.

Dexamethasone is the steroid of choice (Greenberg et al. 1980; Sorensen et al. 1994). It reduces vasogenic edema. Very high doses may be required (100 mg bolus of IV dexamethasone, followed by doses every 6 h of between 4 and 24 mg). It is important to measure the blood glucose of those receiving corticosteroids. Androgen deprivation therapy may be in the form of either radical orchidectomy (which produces a rapid response) or maximal androgen blockade with an antiandrogen combined with an LHRH agonist.

Surgical decompression (laminectomy) is used in patients with a life expectancy of >6 months who have had previous radiotherapy at the involved site, for those whose neurology deteriorates during radiotherapy, or for those who have a cord compression of unknown histology. It is important to ensure compliance with current thromboprophylaxis guidelines and to ensure good care of pressure areas (Rajer and Kovac 2008).

Prognosis

Patients who are still able to walk by the time they receive treatment have a high chance (70–90 %) of remaining ambulatory after treatment. Of those patients who present with complete paralysis prior to onset of treatment, only 20–40 % will regain the ability to walk (Tazi et al. 2003). Of those presenting with urinary retention prior to onset of treatment, only 40 % will regain normal voiding after treatment.

The mean survival of ambulatory patients is longer (on the order of 18 months) compared with those presenting with paraplegia (approximately 4 months) (Smith et al. 1993).

Those patients who have not received androgen deprivation prior to the onset of cord compression survive longer when compared with those who are already on hormone treatment at the time of presentation with cord compression (Huddart et al. 1997; Tazi et al. 2003).

Radiation Cystitis

Pelvic radiation therapy can result in damage to both the urothelium – causing extrusiton of urine from the bladder lumen out through the urothelial layer – and the detrusor muscle resulting in fibrosis and a loss of compliance. The bladder can suffer the after effects of radiation for many years after treatment. The most common symptom is hematuria; this may be in the acute phase or late in presentation. The acute type is usually very soon after treatment, self-limiting, and does not normally require anything beyond conservative management. Hematuria associated with late radiation cystitis has been graded by the European Organization for Research and Treatment of Cancer (EORTC) and the

Grade	Findings
1	Minor telangiectasia (nonvisible hematuria)
2	Generalized telangiectasia (visible hematuria)
3	Severe generalized telangiectasia
4	Severe hemorrhagic cystitis
5	Death from uncontrolled hematuria

Radiation Therapy Oncology Group (RTOG):
Late presentation may occur up to 20 years after treatment, and initial assessment should include the exclusion of infection or recurrent tumor. Initially, the bladder should be irri-

gated and the patient supported with fluid and transfusion as required. Cystodiathermy or laser fulguration may be effective. A wide range of other treatments have been tried; these include oral or parenteral agents such as conjugated estrogens or pentosan polysulfate, with success ranging from 58 to 88 %. Intravesical treatments such aluminum, formalin, or prostaglandins have been used. With a range of success – 50–100 % with aluminum, 71–93 % with formalin – information on prostaglandins is more limited.

The use of a pressurized treatment chamber with 100 % oxygen or hyperbaric oxygen therapy appears to show favorable outcomes (60–92 %) with a very low side-effect profile. The treatment is daily for between 20 and 30 days with sessions lasting up to 2 h (extra time is added for compression and decompression), i.e., a very intense program. But this appears to create beneficial changes such as angiogenesis and fibroblast activity at tissue level. There is need for a randomized study but this remains a sensible treatment option if it is available.

Surgical options may be necessary – interventional radiology may avoid this in some cases with the use of selective embolization. Otherwise, surgical ligation of the internal iliac arteries is one means of stopping bleeding. As the options become progressively invasive, it is sensible to bear in mind that these patients are often complicated and may have other comorbidities. Urinary diversion initially with percutaneous nephrostomies may help or an ileal conduit (with or without cystectomy) is a further surgical option (Smit and Heyns 2010).

Complications of Intravesical Bacillus Calmette-Guerin (BCG)

BCG is used widely in uro-oncology practice for the treatment of high-grade urothelial transitional cell carcinoma. It is a successful treatment but has a significant side-effect profile. These can be classified as local or systemic. In a meta-analysis that looked at 1,471 patients undergoing BCG treatment, there was a 53.8 % incidence of cystitis. Hematuria was found in up to 91 % (Bohle et al. 2003). Epididymitis is also reported (Lamm et al. 2000) with case reports of the need for orchidectomy. The rate is less than 1 %, but there have been reports of a small contracted bladder following BCG treatment. Between 3 and 18 % report systemic symptoms, mostly in the form of fevers. There were no deaths seen in this study but they have also been reported. Treatment of systemic symptoms or local infective symptoms should be undertaken in close consultation with a microbiologist.

References

Bohle A, Jocham D, Bock PR. Intravesical bacillus Calmette-Guerin versus mitomycin C for superficial bladder cancer: a formal meta-analysis of comparative studies on recurrence and toxicity. J Urol. 2003;169:90–5.

Clarke NW. The management of hormone-relapsed prostate cancer. BJU Int. 2003;92:860–6.

Fallon B, Olney L, Culp DA. Nephrostomy in cancer patients. Br J Urol. 1980;52:237–42.

Greenberg HS, Kim JH, Posner JB. Epidural spinal cord compression from metastatic tumor: results from a new protocol. Ann Neurol. 1980;8:361–6.

Hamdy FC, Williams JL. Use of dexamethasone for ureteric obstruction in advanced prostate cancer: percutaneous nephrostomies can be avoided. Br J Urol. 1995;75:782–5.

Huddart RA, Rajan B, Law M. Spinal cord compression in prostate cancer: treatment outcome and prognostic factors. Radiother Oncol. 1997;44:229–36.

Lamm D, Blumenstein B, Crissman J, et al. Maintenance BCG immunotherapy for Ta, T1 and carcinoma in situ transitional cell carcinoma of the urinary bladder. A randomized Southwest Oncology Group Study. J Urol. 2000;163:1124–9.

Rajer M, Kovac V. Malignant spinal cord compression. Radiol Oncol. 2008;42(1):23–31.

Smit SG, Heyns CF. Management of radiation cystitis. Nat Rev Urol. 2010;7:206–14.

ᴣmith EM, Hampel N, Ruff RL, et al. Spinal cord compression secondary to prostate carcinoma: treatment and prognosis. J Urol. 1993;149:330–3.

Soper JT, Blaszczyk TM, Oke E, et al. Percutaneous nephrostomy in gynecologic oncology patients. Am J Obstet Gynecol. 1988; 158:1126–31.

Sorensen PS, Helweg-Larsen S, Mouridsen H, Hansen HH. Effects of high-dose dexamethasone in carcinomatous metastatic spinal cord compression treated with radiotherapy: a randomised trial. Eur J Cancer. 1994;30A.1:22–7.

Tazi H, Manunta A, Rodriguez A, et al. Spinal cord compression in metastatic prostate cancer. Eur Urol. 2003;44:527–32.

Chapter 10
Pediatric Emergencies

Dan Wood

Introduction

Many of the scenarios discussed in the section are not truly emergencies – there are some and they are highlighted. However, the importance of good clinical care and an early understanding for parents is very important and can allay much anxiety – this will improve the lives of the parents, the patient, and those delivering care. Almost all of these topics could be the subject of a chapter or a whole book in their own right. For the purposes of this book, detailed explanations are not included but a summary of core principles. The interested reader should refer to a definitive text on pediatric urology for more detail.

D. Wood, Ph.D., FRCS (Urol)
Department of Adolescent and Reconstructive Urology,
University College London Hospitals,
London, UK

Department of Urology, Great Ormond Street Hospital,
London, UK

University College London,
London, UK
e-mail: dan.wood@uclh.nhs.uk

H. Hashim et al. (eds.), *Urological Emergencies*
In Clinical Practice, DOI 10.1007/978-1-4471-2720-8_10,
© Springer-Verlag London 2013

The Exstrophy-Epispadias Complex

Bladder exstrophy (BE) occurs 1 in every 30,000–50,000 live births (M:F 3:1). A failure of the cloacal membrane results in an undeveloped lower anterior abdominal wall, with an open bladder and bladder neck extruding from the defect, an epispadic penis, and an incomplete pelvic ring resulting in a pubic diastasis. Primary epispadias – where the urethra opens onto the dorsal aspect of the penis – is less common with an incidence of 1:120,000 (M:F 5:1) and does not involve the bladder. The bladder neck may be incontinent; this often correlates with position of the urethral opening – the more proximal, the more likely incontinence will exist. Cloacal exstrophy is a more complex variant of bladder exstrophy that involves an additional failure of separation from the hindgut.

All have their own complexities in terms of reconstruction and long-term management. In the UK, there are two designated centers for the treatment of exstrophy – Royal Manchester Children's Hospital and Great Ormond Street Hospital in London. The rarity and complex nature of these disorders led to a decision that patients would benefit from a concentration of expertise delivered in this way.

Children born with bladder exstrophy are rarely affected by other health problems – in that sense they can be treated normally after delivery and do not require immediate intervention. Eighty percent of boys and 15 % of girls have inguinal herniae, but these may not be recognized at the initial assessment. Vitamin K should be given especially to those having early surgery. The bladder plate should be covered with cling film inside a nappy. Transfer to a center with appropriate expertise needs to follow this – delay by a few hours is acceptable if it means the parents can safely travel with the child. Unless there are other concerns or complications, there is no need for intravenous access or antibiotics prior to transfer. Initial closure of the bladder is ideally performed within the first 48 h of life. This will be preceded by assessment including an ultrasound at the receiving center.

The bladder plate is closed and if possible the diastasis is bought together (the infant pelvis will usually allow this without a need for osteotomies) – facilitating approximation of the rectus muscle and skin. Some centers will attempt a full and definitive reconstruction at this initial stage; other centers opt for a staged approach – the subtleties of each are beyond the needs of this text (Cuckow 2008).

Disorders of Sex Development (DSD)

Broad consultation has led to a change in the use of terms for this complex group of disorders. The banner of "intersex" has been replaced by "disorders of sex development." A clinical means of describing the range of disorders is largely obsolete now but fits well with the reviewed terminology and helps to give a logical way of considering these patients (see Table 10.1). The new terminology allows a more pathological understanding of the underlying disorders and removes some of the more pejorative elements of historical terminology.

The contributing factors to sex development and thus to disorders of the same are:

- Chromosomal (Chromosomal DSD)
- Gonadal development (Gonadal DSD)
- Hormone/receptor synthesis or interaction (Phenotypic/anatomical DSD)

All patients thought to be affected should be discussed and referred to a center with appropriate expertise as soon as

TABLE 10.1 Clinical description along with accepted terminology

Clinical description	Accepted terminology
Under-virilized male	46 XY DSD
Over-virilized female	46 XX DSD
True hermaphrodite	Ovotesticular DSD
Mixed gonadal dysgenesis	Mixed gonadal dysgenesis

possible. Advice can be taken about the timing and location of investigations. These centers should have a multidisciplinary team of experts providing a service for these patients.

Congenital adrenal hyperplasia is the most common cause of 46 XX DSD and accounts for about 85 % of all infants with ambiguous genitalia in the Western world. The immediate medical concern for these patients is life-threatening salt loss. Evaluation of plasma electrolytes and consultation with a pediatric endocrinology service is vital.

The parents should be advised and supported throughout initial assessment and transfer. On arrival in a specialist center, a detailed explanation can be offered about the potential course of investigation. The parents should be told to avoid registering the birth and sex of the child until advised to do so.

Initial history should include family history, including previous DSD, genital anomalies and parental consanguinity, previous neonatal deaths, primary amenorrhoea or infertility in other family members, maternal androgen exposure, and systemic symptoms of the neonate. Physical examination should include the phallus – looking for hypospadias and size, presence of a urogenital sinus, palpable gonads – including site, size, and symmetry and blood pressure. Initial investigations will be 17-hydroxyprogesterone, electrolytes, luteinizing hormone (LH), follicle-stimulating hormone (FSH), testosterone (TST), cortisol, adrenocorticotrophic hormone (ACTH), sex hormone-binding globulin (SHBG), and inhibin-B. A further tests may include urine steroid profile, karyotype, ultrasound, examination under anesthetic ± a genitogram (this is still advocated in guidelines but is not used routinely in all centers), some will prefer an MRI, androgen-binding studies, and an hCG stimulation test.

Gender assignment decisions can be very difficult, and many factors may influence the final choice. A number of medical factors should be accounted for such as:

- Age at presentation
- Fertility potential
- Size of the penis
- Presence of a functional vagina
- Endocrine function
- Malignancy potential
- Antenatal testosterone exposure

- General appearance
- Psychosocial well-being and a stable gender identity (taken from Tekgül et al. 2012)

The family may have major cultural reasons for a particular decision, or psychological barriers have encountered such a difficult situation. These issues need to be worked through with a psychologist and others, all of whom are experts in this field. At times, the team may take ethical advice if decisions seem particularly difficult (Creighton 2013).

Neurogenic Bladder

The management of the neurogenic bladder in pediatric practice has been revolutionized by intermittent catheterization (IC), and this is now the mainstay of treatment in early life. In combination with anticholinergic medication, IC results in improved upper tract outcomes, better bladder preservation, improved long-term continence, and a reduced need for cystoplasty. Parents should be taught IC for their infant as soon as possible, this makes it easier for them to master and improves acceptance by their child as they grow.

Medications used in this group are most commonly oxybutynin, but others including tolterodine, propiverine, and solifenacin have been used.

Careful monitoring of the upper tracts and bladder function with urodynamics are essential to understand both bladder and sphincter function.

Hydronephrosis

Dilatation of the upper urinary tract, or hydronephrosis, is a finding that causes initial alarm among parents and prospective parents. Causes of dilatation may be:

- Obstruction
- Reflux
- Developmental abnormality
- High urine flow

It can be surprisingly difficult to differentiate between these. The importance of this section is to give some safe principles by which to manage the initial presentation.

Obstruction is most sensibly defined as any obstruction to urinary outflow leading to a reduction in renal function.

Indications for intervention will be based on the severity of dilatation – the normal antero-posterior (AP) diameter of the renal pelvis should be no more than 6 mm – and reduction in renal function. Other indications include recurrent urinary tract infections.

Antenatal Diagnosis

A normal dating scan at 16–18 weeks will routinely show the kidneys – the ideal time for visualization of the urinary tract is around 28 weeks of gestation. If hydronephrosis is reported on either scan, other important parameters (severity of dilatation, uni- or bilateral, involvement of the ureter, bladder emptying and volume, sex of the child, and amniotic fluid volume) will give an indication of severity and potentially, diagnosis.

Postnatal Management

In severely affected cases, a repeat ultrasound should be immediate. However, a neonate has a transitory, physiological dehydration that lasts approximately 48 h – a postnatal ultrasound should be organized after this time in less urgent cases. If there is no dilatation at this time, a repeat scan 4 weeks later is recommended (Tekgül 2012). If valves or another form of infravesical obstruction is suspected, early drainage is vital – this is usually possible with an infant feeding tube passed urethrally. If there is difficulty, a suprapubic catheter under ultrasound guidance may be necessary.

For those with persistent hydronephrosis, the list of potential differential diagnoses includes pelvi-ureteric junction (PUJ) obstruction, vesicoureteric junction (VUJ) obstruction, vesicoureteric reflux, posterior urethral valves, ureteroceles, diverticulae, and neurogenic bladder. Up to 25 % may have reflux and a micturating cystourethrogram (MCUG) is the most sensitive way to diagnose this and is still regarded as the gold standard. However, this should be discussed with the parents as the clinical significance of reflux in isolation may be very minor and an MCUG is a very invasive investigation – see Table 10.2 showing the grading of reflux and its rate of spontaneous resolution. In a male infant with bilateral hydronephrosis, it is an essential investigation to assess for valves. In cases with only hydronephrosis and no ureteric involvement, it may not be necessary.

TABLE 10.2 Describing reflux by grade, relative incidence, and rates of spontaneous resolution (RP – renal pelvis) (Tekgül 2012)

Grade of reflux	Description	Incidence of grade (%)	Spontaneous resolution (%)
I	Reflux does not reach RP	7	83
II	Reflux reaches RP, no dilatation of collecting system. Normal fornices	53	60
III	Mild or moderate ureteric dilatation, ± kinking; moderately dilated collecting system; normal or minimally deformed fornices	32	46
IV	Moderate ureteric dilatation ± kinking; moderate dilatation of the collecting system; blunt fornices, papillae still visible	6	9
V	Gross dilatation and kinking of the ureter, marked dilatation of the collecting system; papillary impressions no longer visible; intraparenchymal reflux	2	0

Description from the International Reflux Study Committee

Diuretic renography – most commonly a MAG-3 reno-gram performed under conditions of good hydration and catheterization is key in determining obstruction and differential function. The relative advantages of other forms of scintigraphy are beyond the scope of this chapter but should be discussed with the nuclear medicine department on a case-by-case basis if doubt exists (Thomas 1998, 2008).

Intervention

Important principles apply across all diagnoses – firstly, preservation of renal function is a prime objective; this will come in the form of relief of obstruction and avoidance of infection. Infection may be avoided by the use of prophylactic antibiotics – most often trimethoprim (2 mg/kg/day); there is controversy about this, and some argue that individual infections should be treated rather than using prophylaxis. Studies suggest no difference between the two strategies, but many continue to use prophylaxis. Avoiding constipation is important along with good bladder management. In boys with abnormal urinary tracts, some centers will offer circumcision on the basis of a meta-analysis showing a reduction in urinary tract infections – the number needed to treat was high at 111, but the data support this approach (Singh-Grewal 2005).

Further treatment will vary enormously depending on the diagnosis. In essence, an obstruction will be alleviated either by:

- Reconstruction – e.g., pyeloplasty for a PUJO, ureteric reimplantation of an obstructed ureter or valve ablation
- Drainage – urethral catheter or diversion above the level of obstruction, e.g., ureterostomy or vesicostomy, with a view to stabilization.

Reflux may need treatment if high-grade or if associated with severe, recurrent urinary tract infections. The Pediatric Health Information system in the United States showed that the availability of endoscopic treatments has lead to an increase in intervention for reflux but no increase in open surgery rates. Treatment of low-grade reflux is regarded by some as unnecessary, while others argue that a day case procedure can avoid prolonged use of prophylactic antibiotics. Where possible, a conservative strategy is reasonable followed by endoscopic injection of a bulking agent to the ureteric orifice. In severe forms or where endoscopic injection has failed and bladder dysfunction has been tackled, open reimplantation is necessary.

Posterior Urethral Valves (PUV)

These are found in 1 in 5000 live male births – there is no established familial pattern. Antenatal hydronephrosis is possible from about 14 weeks (though the majority are diagnosed later) and about 80 % of cases are detected on antenatal ultrasound. The early age at detection and oligohydramnios are both indicators of a poor long-term prognosis. Features of an antenatal ultrasound suggestive of PUV are:

- Bilateral hydroureteronephrosis
- Thick-walled bladder (may not seem to empty)
- Dilated posterior urethra
- Oligohydramnios

These features may be replicated on a postnatal ultrasound but an MCUG will provide the definitive diagnosis (see Fig. 10.1). Initial assessment needs to include electrolytes and serum renal function (the first 48 h of measurements will reflect the maternal creatinine). Some have advocated intrauterine treatment with a vesico-amniotic shunt; current guidance suggests that this should only be performed in a specialist center as part of a research program. Once the child is born, bladder drainage is vital – for most an infant feeding passed through the urethra will achieve this – if this is not possible, an ultrasound-guided suprapubic catheter can be placed.

Following MCUG, cystoscopy will confirm the presence of valves and these can then be ablated – there are a variety of

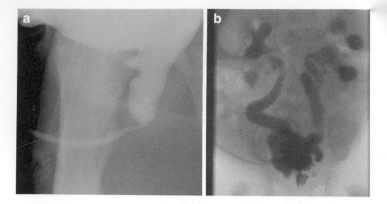

FIGURE 10.1 Micturating cystograms from (**a**) late presenting 15-year-old boy showing the dilated posterior urethra and (**b**) an infant showing dilated posterior urethra, including reflux into the prostatic ducts, very abnormal bladder, and bilateral vesicoureteric reflux

techniques with little to tell between them. The practice most familiar to the author is the use of a cold knife on a pediatric resectoscope with a repeat MCUG at 3 months, a circumcision, and relook cystoscopy to ensure complete resection.

These boys all need long-term follow-up. Data suggest that renal deterioration may continue late into adult life – recognition and treatment are important and may be a means of minimizing further loss of function. Bladder function may also deteriorate with age and needs careful monitoring as part of follow-up. Those looking after these patients in pediatric practice need to ensure safe transition to the care of an "interested" adolescent or adult urologist (Holmdahl 2005).

Urinary Tract Infections (UTI)

In the first year of life, about 4 % of boys and 2 % of girls will have a UTI, and in older prepubertal children, 3 % of girls and 1 % of boys are affected. UTIs should be classified according to site and severity for initial treatment. Other factors may be important in later assessment. Seventy-five percent of infections contain *E. coli.*

Any child presenting with a fever above 38 °C should have a urine culture sent – a clean catch is ideal – otherwise, suprapubic aspiration is an option.

The two key sites are the bladder (cystitis – with symptoms including dysuria, frequency, hematuria, enuresis, and suprapubic pain) and the upper tracts (pyelonephritis – fever, flank pain, tenderness). Severity can be gauged by the degree of fever – with a fever above 39 °C classified as severe and other systemic symptoms such as vomiting or diarrhea making the classification severe.

A full history including questions about poor urinary flow, constipation, recurrent infections, antenatal renal diagnoses, and family history of VUR should be asked. Any child younger than 3 months of age with a UTI should be referred to a pediatric specialist.

All children with pyelonephritis should be referred to a pediatric specialist and treated with 7–10 days of oral antibiotics unless these cannot be taken. Cystitis in those older than 3 months may not need referral unless it recurs. Asymptomatic bacteriuria should not be treated.

Antibiotic prophylaxis is not recommended after a single UTI.

Once treated, parents need to be advised about the importance of a good daily fluid intake and regular voiding.

Current recommendations for imaging suggest that for those younger than 6 months, an ultrasound is indicated acutely if the UTI is complicated or recurrent – this should be followed by an interval DMSA nuclear medicine scan to assess scarring and split function and a MCUG to establish a cause. A straightforward UTI may need an ultrasound, but this can be deferred until the child has recovered. For a single UTI that responds to treatment in 48 h, no imaging is necessary in older children. The use of DMSA is also far more sparing and MCUG is only indicated under specific circumstances such as dilatation on ultrasound, family history of VUR, poor urine flow or a non-E. coli infection (NICE guideline 54 2007).

It is important that parents know what triggers should bring them back, but the most straightforward cases will not need follow-up.

References

Creighton SM, Wood D. Complex gynaecological and urological problems in adolescents: challenges and transition. Postgrad Med J. 2013;89(1047):34–8. doi: 10.1136/postgradmedj-2012-131232.

Cuckow PM. Bladder exstrophy and epispadias. In: Duffy PG, Thomas DFM, Rickwood AMK, editors. Essentials of paediatric urology. 2nd ed. London: Informa; 2008. ISBN 1-84184-633-3.

Holmdahl G, Sillen U. Boys with posterior urethral valves: outcomes concerning renal function, bladder function and paternity at ages 31 to 44. J Urol. 2005;174:1031–4.

NICE guideline 54. UTI in children. 2007. http://www.nice.org.uk/nicemedia/live/11819/36032/36032.pdf.

Singh-Grewal D, Macdessi J, Craig J. Circumcision for the prevention of urinary tract infection in boys: a systematic review of randomised trials and observational studies. Arch Dis Child. 2005;90(8):853–8.

Tekgül S, Riedmiller H, Dogan HS, Gerharz E, Hoebeke P, Kocvara R, Nijman R, Radmayr Chr, Stein R. Paediatric urology. EAU Guidelines. 2012.

Thomas DF. Prenatally detected uropathy: epidemiological considerations. Br J Urol. 1998;81 Suppl 2:8–12.

Thomas DF. Upper tract obstruction. In: Duffy PG, Thomas DFM, Rickwood AMK, editors. Essentials of paediatric urology. 2nd ed. London: Informa; 2008. ISBN 1-84184-633-3.

Chapter 11
Common Emergency Urological Procedures

John Reynard and Nigel C. Cowan

Urethral Catheterization

Indications

Indications for urethral catheterization include relief of urinary retention; prevention of urinary retention—a period of postoperative catheterization is commonly employed after many operations where limited mobility makes normal voiding difficult; monitoring of urine output, e.g., postoperatively; prevention of damage to the bladder during cesarean section;

J. Reynard, DM, FRCS (Urol) (✉)
Department of Urology, Nuffield Department of Surgical Sciences,
Oxford University Hospitals, Oxford, UK

The National Spinal Injuries Centre, Stoke Mandeville Hospital,
Aylesbury, UK
e-mail: john.reynard@ouh.nhs.uk

N.C. Cowan, M.A., MB, BChir, FRCR
Department of Radiology, The Churchill Hospital,
Oxford, UK
e-mail: nigel.cowan@radiology.oxford.ac.uk

H. Hashim et al. (eds.), *Urological Emergencies*
In Clinical Practice, DOI 10.1007/978-1-4471-2720-8_11,
© Springer-Verlag London 2013

bladder drainage following surgery to the bladder, prostate, or urethra, e.g., transurethral resection of the prostate (TURP), transurethral resection of bladder tumor (TURBT), open bladder stone removal, and radical prostatectomy; and bladder drainage following injuries to the bladder.

Technique

Explain the need for and method of catheterization to the patient. Use the smallest catheter—in practical terms usually a 12 Ch, with a 10-mL balloon. For longer catheterization periods (weeks), use a Silastic catheter to limit tissue reaction, thereby reducing risk of a catheter-induced urethral stricture. If you suspect clot retention (a history of hematuria prior to the episode of retention), use a three-way catheter (20 Ch or greater) to allow evacuation of clots and bladder irrigation to prevent subsequent catheter blockage.

The technique is aseptic. One gloved hand is sterile; the other is "dirty." The dirty hand holds the penis or separates the labia to allow cleansing of the urethral meatus; this hand should not touch the catheter. Use sterile water or sterile cleaning solution to "prep" the skin around the meatus.

Apply lubricant jelly to the urethra. Traditionally, this contains local anesthetic [e.g., 2 % lignocaine (lidocaine)], which takes between 3 and 5 min to work. However, a randomized placebo-controlled trial showed that 2 % lignocaine was no more effective for pain relief than anesthetic-free lubricant (Birch et al. 1994), suggesting that it is the lubricant action that prevents urethral pain. If using local anesthetic lubricant, warn the patient that it may "sting." Local anesthetic lubricant is contraindicated in patients with allergies to local anesthetics and in those with urethral trauma, where there is a (theoretical) risk of complications arising from systemic absorption of lignocaine. When instilling the lubricant jelly, do so gently, as a sudden, forceful depression of plunger of syringe can rupture the urethra! In males, "milk" the gel toward the posterior urethra while squeezing the meatus to prevent it from coming back out of the meatus.

Insert the catheter using the sterile hand, until flow of urine confirms it is in the bladder. Failure of urine flow may indicate that the catheter balloon is in the urethra. Intraurethral inflation of the balloon can rupture the urethra. Do not inflate the balloon if no urine flows! If no urine flows, attempt aspiration of urine using a 50-mL bladder syringe (lubricant gel can occlude eyeholes of catheter). Absence of urine flow indicates either that the catheter is not in the bladder or, if the indication for the catheterization is retention, that the diagnosis is wrong (there will usually be a few milliliters of urine in the bladder even in cases where the absence of micturition is due to oliguria or anuria, so complete absence of urine flow usually indicates the catheter is not in the bladder). If the catheter will not pass into the bladder and you are sure that the patient is in retention, proceed with suprapubic catheterization.

Suprapubic Catheterization

Indications

Indications are failed urethral catheterization in urinary retention; preferred site for long-term catheters.

Long-term *urethral* catheters commonly lead to acquired hypospadias in males (ventral splitting of glans penis) and a patulous urethra in females (leading to frequent balloon expulsion and bypassing of urine around the catheter). Hence, the suprapubic site is preferred for long-term catheters.

Contraindications

Suprapubic catheterization is best avoided in (1) patients with clot retention, the cause of which may be an underlying bladder cancer (the cancer could be spread along the catheter track to involve the skin); (2) patients with lower midline incisions (bowel may be "stuck" to the deep aspect of the scar, leading to the potential for bowel perforation); and (3) pelvic fractures, where the catheter may inadvertently enter the large pelvic hematoma, which always accompanies severe pelvic fracture. This can lead to infection of the hematoma, and the resulting sepsis can be fatal! Failure to pass a urethral catheter in a patient with a pelvic fracture usually indicates a urethral rupture (confirmed by urethrography) and is an indication for formal open, suprapubic cystotomy.

Technique

Prior to insertion of the trocar, be sure to confirm the diagnosis by (a) abdominal examination (palpate and percuss the lower abdomen to confirm the bladder is distended), (b) ultrasound (in practice usually not available), and (c) aspiration of urine (using a green needle). Patients with lower abdominal scars may have bowel interposed between the abdominal wall and bladder, and this can be perforated if the trocar is inserted near the scar and without prior aspiration of urine! In such cases, ultrasound-guided catheterization may be sensible.

Use a wide-bore trocar if you anticipate that the catheter will be in place for more than 24 h (small-bore catheters will block within a few days). Aim to place the catheter about two to three fingerbreadths above the pubis symphysis. Placement too close to the symphysis will result in difficult trocar insertion (the trocar will hit the symphysis). Instill a few milliliters of local anesthetic into the skin of the intended puncture site and down to the rectus sheath. Confirm the location of the bladder by drawing back on the needle to aspirate urine from the bladder. This helps guide the angle of trocar insertion. Make a 1-cm incision with a sharp blade through the skin. Hold the trocar handle in your right hand (if you are right-handed), and steady the needle end with your left hand (this hand helps prevent insertion too deeply). Push the trocar in the same direction in which you previously aspirated urine. As soon as urine issues from the trocar, push the trocar further down by about 1–2 cm and withdraw the latter, holding the attached sheath in place. Make sure you do not push the trocar through the posterior bladder wall. Push the catheter in as far as it will go. Inflate the balloon. Peel away the side of the sheath and remove it.

British Association of Urological Surgeons' Suprapubic Catheter (SPC) Practice Guidelines 2010 (Harrison et al. 2010)

- If appropriate expertise for SPC insertion is not available, suprapubic aspiration of urine using a needle up to 21G can be used as a temporary measure to temporarily relieve the patient's retention.
- Use regional or general anesthesia if the bladder cannot be comfortably filled with at least 300 mL of fluid.
- Use antibiotic prophylaxis.
- Ultrasound may be used. "However, the practitioner involved must have appropriate training and experience. Ultrasonography should only be used to look for interposing bowel loops along the planned catheter track by individuals who have received specific training and are experienced in this task" ("appropriate training and experience" are not defined by BAUS).
- It is reasonable to use a closed technique where the bladder is readily palpable and there is no history of lower abdominal surgery, providing urine can be easily aspirated from the bladder using a needle passed along the planned catheter track.
- Where the bladder cannot be palpated, blind insertion should not be undertaken.

- Where there is a history of lower abdominal surgery, use an open technique or ultrasound to exclude the presence of bowel loops on the intended catheter track.

Bladder Washout for Blocked Catheter

This may be required after TURP or TURBT. Try to avoid the problem by ensuring that the nursing staff is familiar with this potential complication. Nurses should be aware of the importance of keeping the catheter bag empty and ensuring that there is always a sufficient supply of irrigant solution. If the urine collection bag becomes full, urine flow ceases and the catheter can become blocked with clot.

The patient will complain of lower abdominal pain, and the bladder will be distended (dull to percussion and tense to palpation). Look at the irrigation channel of the three-way catheter. There will be no flow of fluid out of the bladder. A small clot may have blocked the catheter or a chip of prostate may have stuck in the eye of the catheter.

Attach a bladder syringe to the end of the catheter and pull back. This may suck out the clot or chip of prostate and flow may restart. If it does not, draw some irrigant up into the syringe until it is about half-full, and forcefully inject this fluid into the bladder. This may dislodge (and fragment) a clot that has stuck to the eye of the catheter. If the problem persists, change the catheter. The obstructing chip of prostate may appear on the end of the catheter as it is withdrawn.

If the bladder is full of clot, then it is sometimes possible, by alternating irrigation and sucking back on the syringe, to remove the clot, but if there is a large quantity in the bladder, you may well have to return the patient to the operating room, remove all the clot by reinserting the resectoscope and applying an Ellik evacuator, and then find and cauterize the bleeding vessel that caused the problem in the first place.

The same technique should be used for post-TURBT catheter blockage as for post-TURP catheter blockage. However, beware of applying over-vigorous pressure to the bladder following resection of a tumor, since the wall of the bladder will have been weakened at the site of tumor resection and it is possible to perforate the bladder. This is particularly so with the thin bladders of elderly women.

Blocked Catheters Following Bladder Augmentation or Neobladder

Again, the suture line of these bladders is weak, and over-vigorous irrigation with a bladder syringe can rupture the bladder. Gently fill the bladder with a 100 mL or so of saline, and very gently wash this fluid around the bladder with the syringe. This can help to dilute a mucus plug allowing sponta-neous flow to be reestablished.

JJ Stent Insertion

Indications in Urological Emergencies

Obstructing ureteric stones
Ureteric injury
Malignant obstruction of the ureter

Preparation of the Patient for JJ Stent Insertion

Oral ciprofloxacin 250 mg; lignocaine gel for urethral anes-thesia and lubrication; sedoanalgesia (diazemuls 2.5–10 mg i.v., pethidine 50–100 mg i.v.). Monitor pulse and oxygen satu-ration with a pulse oximeter.

Technique

A flexible cystoscope is passed into the bladder and rotated through 180°. This allows greater deviation of the end of the cystoscope and makes identification of the ureteric orifice easier. A 0.9-mm hydrophilic guidewire (Terumo

266 J. Reynard and N.C. Cowan

Corporation, Japan) is passed into the ureter under direct vision (Fig. 11.1a). The guidewire is manipulated into the renal pelvis using C-arm digital fluoroscopy (Fig. 11.1b). The cystoscope is placed close to the ureteric orifice, and its position relative to bony landmarks in the pelvis is recorded by frame-grabbing a fluoroscopic image. The flexible cystoscope is then removed and a 4-Ch ureteric catheter is passed over the guidewire into the renal pelvis. A small quantity of

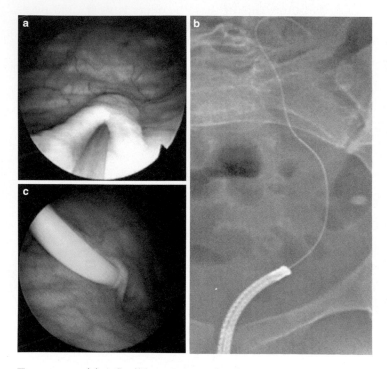

FIGURE 11.1 (a) A flexible cystoscope has been passed into the bladder and a guidewire is manipulated into the ureter under direct vision. (See this figure in full color in the insert.) (b) Under fluoroscopic control, the guidewire is advanced up the ureter and into the renal pelvis. (c) The lower end of the stent is seen deployed in the bladder. (See this figure in full color in the insert.) (d) Previously instilled contrast medium can be used to confirm that the stent is in the correct position

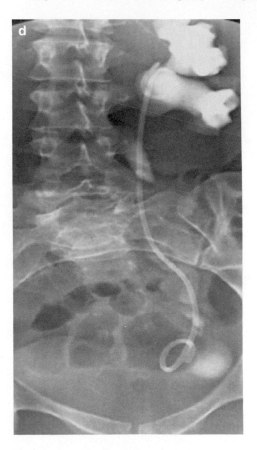

FIGURE 11.1 (continued)

nonionic contrast medium is injected into the renal collecting system to outline its position and to dilate it. The Terumo guidewire is replaced with an ultra-stiff guidewire (Cook UK Ltd., Letchworth, UK), and the 4-Ch ureteric catheter is removed. We use a variety of stent sizes depending on the patient's size (6–8 Ch, 20–26 cm) (Boston Scientific Ltd., St. Albans, UK). The stent is advanced to the renal pelvis under fluoroscopic control, checking that the lower end of the stent is not inadvertently pushed up the ureter by checking the position of the ureteric orifice on the previously frame-grabbed image (Fig. 11.1c). The guidewire is then removed (Fig. 11.1d).

Percutaneous Nephrostomy Insertion

Indications in Urological Emergencies

- Pyonephrosis (infected hydronephrosis)
- Obstruction due to ureteric stone (JJ stent preferable)
- Obstructive renal failure (e.g., bilateral ureteric obstruction from locally advanced prostate cancer)

Preparation of the Patient for Nephrostomy Insertion

Patients should have their blood clotting checked, and serum should be grouped and saved in case heavy bleeding occurs, and blood transfusion is required. Verbal consent should be taken and the discussion about risks documented in the patient's notes (see section Complications).

Technique

This procedure is performed under local anesthetic with or without sedation and with antibiotic cover (depending on urine culture; cefuroxime and gentamicin if no culture result is available). The patient lies prone. A nephrostomy needle is inserted into the renal pelvis and contrast is instilled to outline the collecting system of the kidney (Fig. 11.2a). A guidewire is passed into the renal pelvis (Fig. 11.2b), and over this, the nephrostomy tube is advanced (Fig. 11.2c).

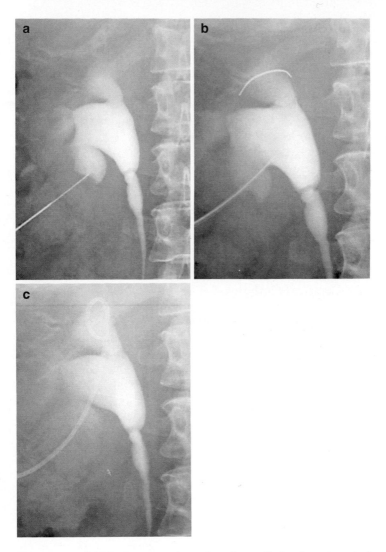

FIGURE 11.2 (**a**) Nephrostomy insertion. A needle has been inserted into the renal pelvis and contrast has been instilled. (**b**) A guidewire has been passed into the renal pelvis. (**c**) The nephrostomy tube is advanced over the guidewire into the renal pelvis

Complications

These will depend on how experienced the radiologist is and on how many nephrostomies he or she inserts per year. The complication rate of dedicated uro-radiologists is lower than that which is generally regarded as acceptable (Ramchandani et al. 2001). Quoted complication rates should be those relevant to your hospital.

In the UK, acceptable complication rates are hemorrhage requiring embolization or surgery 1 %, septic shock 4 %, damage to adjacent organs <1 %, and failure to drain the kidney approximately 5 % (Ramchandani et al. 2001), but some series report complication rates that are below these (Ho and Cowan 2002).

Failure to Deflate Catheter Balloon for Removal of a Urethral Catheter

From time to time, an inflated catheter balloon will not deflate when the time comes for removal of the catheter. No amount of drawing back on the balloon channel with a syringe will make the balloon go down, and attempts to burst the balloon by inflating the balloon with air or flushing the balloon inflation channel with water fail to work.

A little patience is required. Leave a 10-mL syringe firmly inserted in the balloon channel, and come back an hour or so later. Sometimes, for no apparent reason, the balloon will have deflated and the catheter will be lying in the bed, having fallen out.

If this does not work and the patient is female, then it is quite easy to burst the balloon using a needle introduced alongside your finger into the vagina (Fig. 11.3). Ask the patient to lie on her back; place a needle on your finger, apply copious lubrication, and gently insert the finger into the vagina. Pull down on the catheter with your other hand (or ask an assistant to do so), until you can feel the balloon of the catheter sitting at the bladder neck. By pulling the balloon onto the needle (which should be advanced a little so it

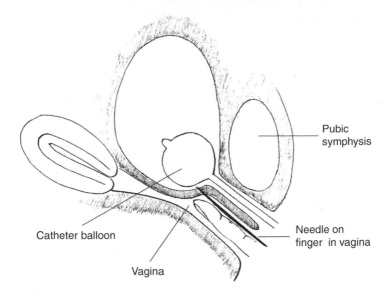

Pubic
symphysis

Catheter balloon

Needle on
finger in vagina

Vagina

FIGURE 11.3 Technique for bursting a catheter balloon in a woman

advances just beyond the tip of your finger), the balloon can be deflated.

In male patients, balloon deflation with a needle can also be done, but ultrasound-guided balloon puncture will be required.

Either the catheter should be clamped to allow the bladder to fill up or the bladder can be filled with saline using a bladder syringe. As the bladder is so inflated, the bowel is pushed upward, out of harm's way, so that the needle can be introduced percutaneously and directly, by ultrasound, toward the balloon of the catheter.

References

Birch BRP, Ratan P, Morley R, et al. Flexible cystoscopy in men: is topical anaesthesia with lignocaine gel worthwhile? Br J Urol. 1994;73:155–9.

Harrison SCW, Lawrence WT, Morley R, et al. British Association of Urological Surgeons' suprapubic catheter practice guidelines. Br J Urol Int. 2010;107:77–85.

Hellawell GO, Cowan NC, Holt SJ, Mutch SJ. A radiation perspective for treating loin pain in pregnancy by double-pigtail stents. Br J Urol Int. 2002;90:801–8.

Ho S, Cowan NC, Holt SJ, et al. Percutaneous nephrostomy (PCN): preliminary results from a prospective pilot study. Eur J Radiol. 2002;12:D3.

McFarlane J, Cowan N, Holt S, Cowan M. Outpatient ureteric procedures: a new method for retrograde ureteropyelography and ureteric stent placement. Br J Urol Int. 2001;87:172–6.

Ramchandani P, et al. Quality improvement guidelines for percutaneous nephrostomy. J Vasc Interv Radiol. 2001;12:1247–51.

Index

H. Hashim et al. (eds.), *Urological Emergencies In Clinical Practice,* DOI 10.1007/978-1-4471-2720-8,
© Springer-Verlag London 2013